simply®

chakras

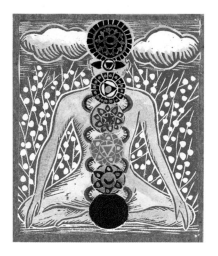

simply ®

chakras

SASHA FENTON

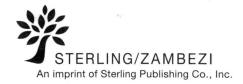

STERLING/ZAMBEZI

An imprint of Sterling Publishing Co., Inc.

New York / London

www.sterlingpublishing.com

STERLING and the distinctive Sterling logo are registered
trademarks of Sterling Publishing Co., Inc.

Library of Congress Cataloging-in-Publication Data

Fenton, Sasha.
  Simply chakras / Sasha Fenton.
    p. cm.
  Includes index.
  ISBN 978-1-4027-5458-6
  1. Chakras. I. Title.
  BF1442.C53F46 2009
  131—dc22   2008032405

2   4   6   8   10   9   7   5   3   1

Published by Sterling Publishing Co., Inc.
387 Park Avenue South, New York, NY 10016
Text © 2009 by Sasha Fenton
Chapter opening illustrations © 2009 by Hannah Firmin
All other illustrations © 2009 by Adam Raiti
Published in the UK solely by Zambezi Publishing Ltd,
PO Box 221, Plymouth, PL2 2EQ
Distributed in Canada by Sterling Publishing
c/o Canadian Manda Group, 165 Dufferin Street
Toronto, Ontario, Canada M6K 3H6
Distributed in Australia by Capricorn Link (Australia) Pty. Ltd.
P.O. Box 704, Windsor, NSW 2756, Australia

Printed in China
All rights reserved

Sterling ISBN 978-1-4027-5458-6
Zambezi ISBN 978-1-903065-62-4

For information about custom editions, special sales, premium
and corporate purchases, please contact Sterling Special Sales
Department at 800-805-5489 or specialsales@sterlingpublishing.com.

contents

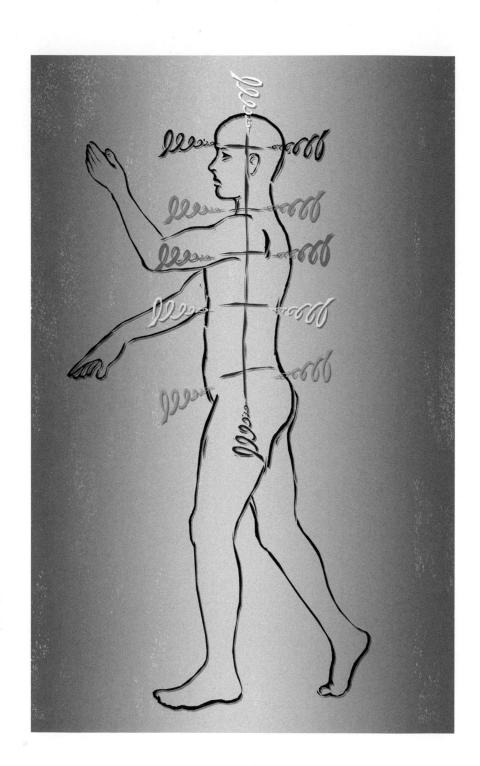

introduction

The word "chakra" derives from a Sanskrit word meaning "wheel" or "disc." Chakras are variously described as spinning vortices, cones, discs, or even cogs. Imagine a length of pipe running through the body with cones that resemble the open ends of trombones sticking out of the front and the back of the body. The pipe-and-cones concept spins. There are seven basic chakras, and each spins in the direction opposite the one previous.

Chakras are said to be part of the human body; they are also said to exist in the bodies of other mammals and possibly of all living creatures. You cannot see chakras on an X-ray or a scan because they are part of a "subtle" energy system, in the same way the aura is. There seem to be links between the chakras and the endocrine system, the nerve ganglia that lie along the spinal column, and the glands that supply us with hormones such as adrenaline, insulin, estrogen, and progesterone.

Chakras are always active; they are constantly monitoring our environment, including light, warmth, sound, smells, tastes, comfort, and discomfort. Chakras relate to the five senses—smell, taste, touch, hearing, and sight—as well as to intuition and spirituality. The chakras sense and measure the elements that surround us, and then balance our bodily interactions with them. The chakras also monitor our interior selves, the basic spiritual elements of fire, earth, air, and water, and work with the human aura to let us know when we are getting too hot, cold, wet, or dry for comfort. They sense when the wind is too strong and perhaps when a rainstorm will come. They are part of the human survival mechanism, and they act as an early warning system. In fact, they may be a very ancient form of survival strategy that exists in all animals and human beings. Chakras also help us to sense and evaluate emotional atmospheres, so if a situation is likely to turn ugly, the chakras alert our sixth sense to tell us to prepare for a fight or to make a run for it.

When a chakra is closed, partially blocked, misaligned, or too open, it throws some part of our health, our personality, or our ability to sense danger off course. I know from my own experience that exhaustion and worry can make me lose perspective, and when this happens, problems that I can normally handle perfectly well suddenly appear overwhelming. When I am overtired or very worried, I forget to eat. When I start to eat again, I might overdo it, or munch on the wrong kind of food.

Now, before you read all about chakras and discover what they mean, take a look at your own body's reactions and see if one or two of the body areas start to "talk" to you. Make a note of the way you react in the following situations.

- When you are too hot, which part of your body perspires most?
- When you get cold, which part of the body feels most chilly?
- Where in your body do you feel joy?
- Where in your body do you feel fear?

- Where in your body do you feel unhappiness?
- What are your weak health points?
- What are your health or bodily strong points?
- What are your strengths? Do you have a kind heart, a good brain, strong muscles, etc.?

Once you discover more about chakras in the chapters to come, you'll know how to respond in positive ways to increase the strength of the chakra that is affected. For example, say that you respond strongly to stressful situations. Your heart no doubt always thumps when you are nervous. Your heart chakra is reacting to the situation. A simple solution is to wear something green whenever you set out to do something challenging. Why? Because this color relates to the heart chakra. (You'll read more about heart chakras in Chapter 7.)

Another example of chakra response would be someone who becomes loud or aggressive under pressure. Such a person would be experiencing a strong response of the base chakra—the chakra at the base of the spine. (For more about this chakra, see Chapter 4.) Red is the color for the base chakra, so this particular person should avoid this color and choose a calming color instead, such as pale blue or light gray.

A strong awareness of your chakras will help you to improve your life and health. So, without further ado, immerse yourself in the amazing system of the chakras and find out what they can do for you.

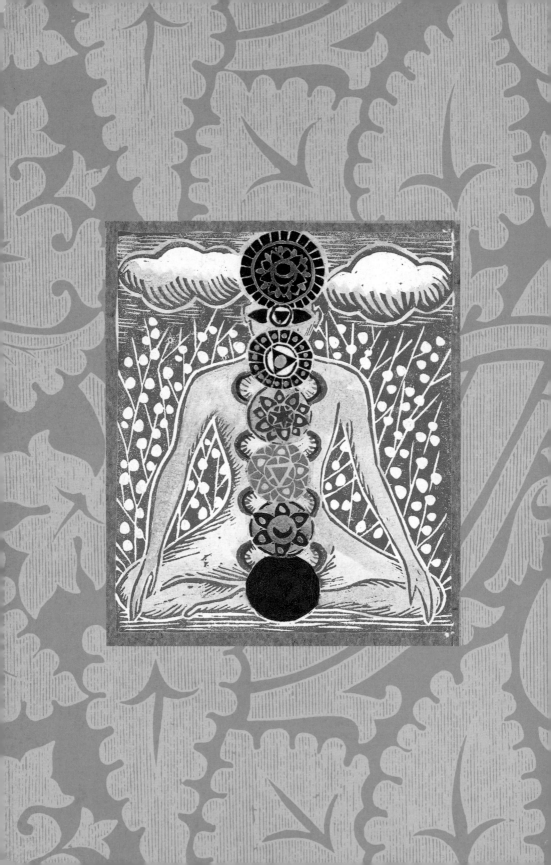

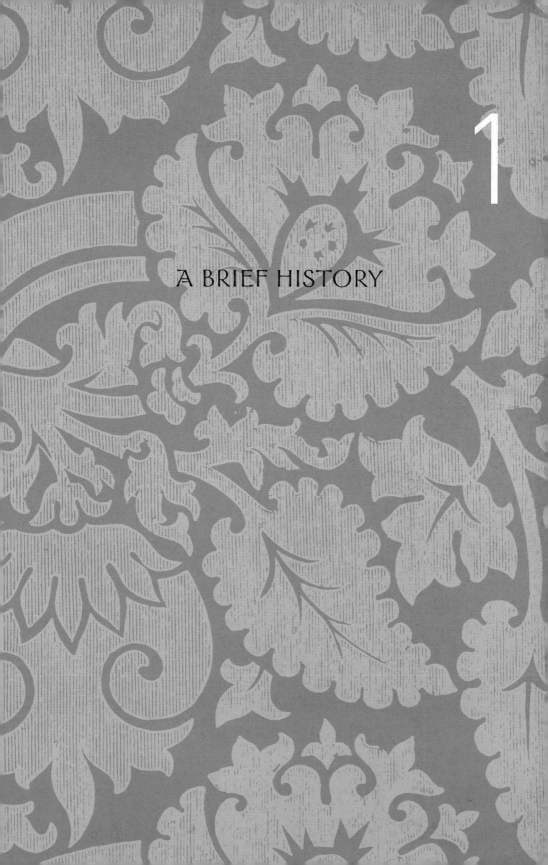

1

A BRIEF HISTORY

The chakra system has its origins in India; its concepts are incorporated into Hinduism and Buddhism. Chakras are mentioned in the Vedas, four holy books that Hindus believe date back to between 1500 and 1200 BC. The earliest mention of the chakras is in the later Upanishads, including the Brahman Upanishad and the Taittiriya Upanishad. This early Vedic model was later adapted into Tibetan Buddhism.

Sir John Woodroffe, who wrote under the name Arthur Avalon, interpreted two early texts called Sat-cakra-nirupana and Paduka-pancaka. He called his book *The Serpent Power*, and the ideas he discussed in it were complex. Later, the Theosophists took an interest in the book and the subject, and in their practice they removed some of the unnecessary complications inherent in Woodroffe's ideas. One of the Theosophists, C. W. Leadbeater, meditated on the subject and then wrote his ideas down in a book called *The Chakras*. Modern Indian scholars have studied Leadbeater's ideas, and they find themselves in broad agreement with him.

In the Vedic (Hindu) tradition, the chakras are linked with the god Vishnu, who is "the Protector of the Universe." Vishnu is linked to the stars, the galaxies, and the universe, so those who have faith in astrology worship him.

Other traditions use systems similar to the chakras, essentially connecting paths around the body; included in these practices is the Chinese system of meridian lines used in acupuncture, along with the related practices of acupressure and reflexology. The aura is another subtle type of

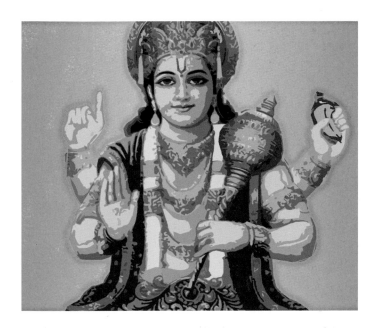

energy, although this may be partially explained in a scientific manner by the electrostatic energy field that surrounds us. There is even some similarity between the chakra system and the Kabala, and even with ideas contained in Islamic Sufism.

In modern times, most of those who tune into subtle vibrations, give energy healing, or channel messages from spirit understand and use the chakra system. Those who meditate know that they must open their chakras before doing so and close down again once they have finished. Interestingly. the chakra system has even had a mention on the *CSI* television program.

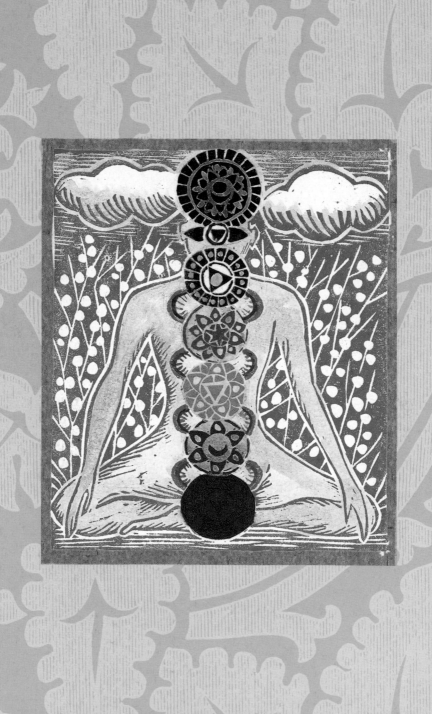

2

ABOUT CHAKRAS

HOW MANY CHAKRAS EXIST?

Not everybody agrees about the total number of chakras or all their locations, but here is a commonly held framework:

- There are seventy-eight thousand chakras in the human body.
- Seven are major chakras.
- Twenty-one are minor chakras.
- Forty-nine are tiny chakras.
- The remainder are minute nano-chakras.

LOTUS FLOWER SYMBOLS

Many Indian illustrations depict the chakras as lotus flowers (water lilies). The number of petals on each flower increases or changes with the growing complexity of each chakra. These artistic renderings do not coordinate with the idea of spinning cones and pipes, so we must understand the flower images as symbolic, probably a way for illiterate people to identify the chakras. Some people confuse these flowers with the chakras themselves, which infuriates purists to the point that they reject the idea of the flower symbols completely. I am a great believer in doing what works for you, so if you wish to imagine the chakras as flowers, please do so. When I first learned about the chakras, my teacher described them to me as common flowers (poppies, marigolds, etc.), so I still remember them that way.

The Hindu Lotus Flower System

Base: Four petals
Sacral: Six petals
Solar plexus: Ten petals
Heart: Twelve petals
Throat: Sixteen petals
Brow: A petal on each side of a
                        circle
Crown: Several violet petals in a
                        flower shape

BASE CHAKRA

THROAT CHAKRA

SACRAL CHAKRA

BROW CHAKRA

SOLAR PLEXUS CHAKRA

CROWN CHAKRA

HEART CHAKRA

Lotus Flower
Designs

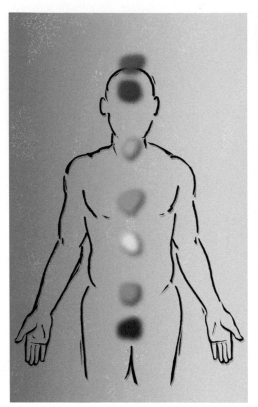

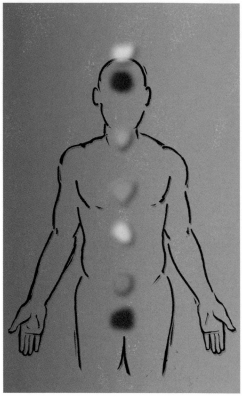

Chakra Color System #1:
Red, Orange, Yellow, Green,
Sky Blue, Indigo, Violet

Chakra Color System #2:
Red, Orange, Yellow, Green,
Sky Blue, Indigo, White

COLORS

When we review the colors used to represent the chakras, we encounter several more discrepancies. Most people believe that the chakras are in the colors of the rainbow, and I have used the standard rainbow system in this book. If you want to assign different colors to the chakras in your practice, please do so; it's important that you work with the techniques that feel right to you.

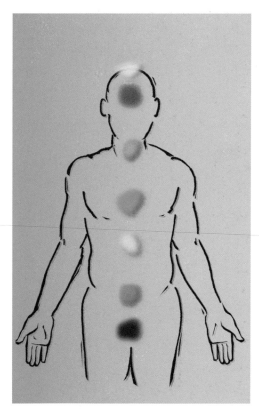

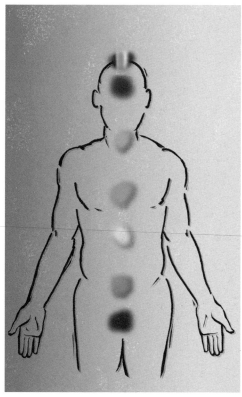

Chakra Color System #3:
Red, Orange, Yellow, Green,
Sky Blue, Violet, White

Chakra Color System #4:
Red, Orange, Yellow, Green,
Sky Blue, Violet, Multicolored

Note: When describing the chakras, I take the traditional route, starting with the base chakra and working upward.

Others use part of the rainbow system but change the color system when they get to the brow and crown chakras. In one case, the brow chakra is indigo and the crown chakra is white; in another, the brow chakra is violet and the crown chakra is white; while yet another tradition makes the upper-most chakra multicolored; and so on.

There is also an eight-chakra system, which uses the usual seven colors of the rainbow and then adds an eighth chakra that is suspended over the head. This system allows for all the usual rainbow colors, plus white.

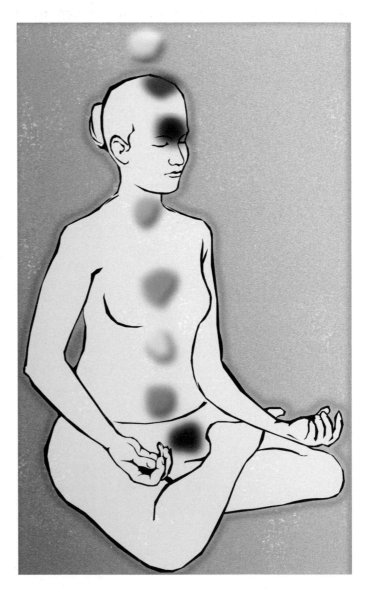

Chakra Color System #5: Red, Orange, Yellow, Green, Sky Blue, Indigo, Violet, White (Eight-Chakra System)

There must have been many different ideas of how to symbolize the chakras over the centuries, but modern psychics often simplify the chakra system to suit modern ideas. There is no hard-and-fast rule, however, because the chakra system will work even if you create a mental design that is entirely your own invention.

CHAKRAS AND ASTROLOGY

Each of the seven chakras is linked to the Sun, the Moon, or one of the five planets (other than Earth) that were known before the invention of the telescope. The signs with which they are linked belong to traditional astrology, as they don't use the "new" planets of Uranus, Neptune and Pluto.

Chakra	Zodiac Sign	Planet
Base	Aries, Scorpio	Mars
Sacral	Cancer	Moon
Solar plexus	Leo	Sun
Heart	Taurus, Libra	Venus
Throat	Gemini, Virgo	Mercury
Brow	Sagittarious, Pisces	Jupiter
Crown	Capricorn, Aquarius	Saturn

LINKED CHAKRAS

If a lower chakra, such as the base, sacral, or solar plexus chakra, is blocked, the upper ones can't work properly. If, for example, the actions of the throat or brow chakra are affected, you may discover that clearing a third chakra, below the throat or brow chakra, helps the affected one to function properly.

OPENING THE CHAKRAS

There are as many methods of opening and closing chakras as there are groups of channelers and healers. The following method comes from my friend, the healer and medium Barbara Ellen, and it uses common international flower images.

Imagine yourself gathering light from the whole universe, and then bringing this light down to the crown chakra. See the crown chakra as a purple lotus (water lily), and imagine it opening and allowing the light to enter through it. Then allow the light to come down as far as the brow chakra, at which point a large blue eye opens. Allow the light to come down as far as the throat chakra, at which point a pale blue cornflower opens. Allow the light to come down to the heart chakra, where a bunch of green leaves opens. Allow the light to come down to the solar plexus chakra and let a large yellow daisy or dahlia open. Allow the light to come down to the solar plexus chakra, where a large orange marigold opens. Allow the light to come down to the base chakra, where a big red poppy opens. Then allow the light to filter down through the legs and to fill the whole body and the surrounding aura. Finish by imagining the light extending down into the earth.

CLOSING THE CHAKRAS

Start by imagining the light that has reached down into the earth being turned off. Then turn off the light in your legs until you reach the base chakra. Now turn off the light there and carefully close the red poppy. Next, turn off the light up to and beyond the solar plexus and close that flower tightly. Continue the process until you have finished, and then send the light off into the universe.

Frankly, it is more important to learn how to close the chakras than open them, because they open of their own volition as soon as you do any kind of psychic or spiritual work. They will also open if you talk or read about psychic matters, or when you watch a psychic or spooky television program. Chakras that have been left open can lead to bad dreams, feelings of psychic invasion, and other uncomfortable sensations.

CLEARING THE CHAKRAS

Life is not always easy, so if you feel overwhelmed or burdened by troubles or if someone or something has upset you, it may be worth clearing the chakras, as doing so can make you feel better. This idea for clearing the chakras comes from Eve Bingham, medium, healer, and secretary of the British Astrological and Psychic Society. Imagine crystal-clear water entering your crown chakra and running through your body and out through your fingertips and toes. Focus

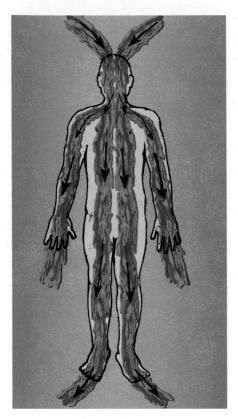

Visualization of
Clearing Chakras
(with Water)

on giving each chakra a good wash. When you have finished, close your chakras carefully.

If you feel that something has really upset you, as soon as you can get around to it, take a shower. While you are under the shower, wash your hair thoroughly, and don't forget to give the bottoms of your feet a good wash. Then perform the chakra-closing procedure again. This can actually help if someone upsets you, because the nastiness will have gotten into your aura, or subtle body, and gotten stuck there like bits of Velcro. A bath will help, but a shower does a better job of washing unwanted subtle material away from the body.

IS CHAKRA WORK HARMFUL?

All psychic work can make the practitioner or the recipient feel light-headed and spacey. If this happens to you, take your shoes off and walk around on the ground, or even lie down on the ground for a while, if possible. As soon as you can do so, go outside and stand on the grass or the earth for a few minutes. This will act like a grounding wire or a lightning conductor, and it will ground you once again.

If you get a headache while giving or receiving healing or performing any other kind of psychic work, stop for a while. The headache denotes too much activity going on in your upper chakras, and a need to ground and balance the lower ones. It might be worth focusing on sending light from your body downward through the earth at this time. Another way to ground yourself might be to lick a little salt or to hold a couple of crystals in your hands, as these items are part of the earth realm.

Always close your chakras after working. If you don't have the time to close them properly, or if you forget how to, this advice from my friend, the medium, healer, and chairman of the British Astrological and Psychic Society, David Bingham, will do the trick. Imagine yourself in a purple sleeping bag, zipped up all around you, and even over your head. You only need to do this for a minute for it to strengthen your aura.

GIVING THINGS UP

Some people believe that those who work with chakras should never touch alcohol and that they should be strictly vegan. These opinions are extreme and unnecessary. However, while there's no need to go to such extremes in your everyday life, it is not easy to perform any kind of psychic or healing work on a very full stomach or when one is tipsy or unwell, so try to maintain a healthy lifestyle, and save the glass of wine for a time when you won't be engaging in psychic or healing work.

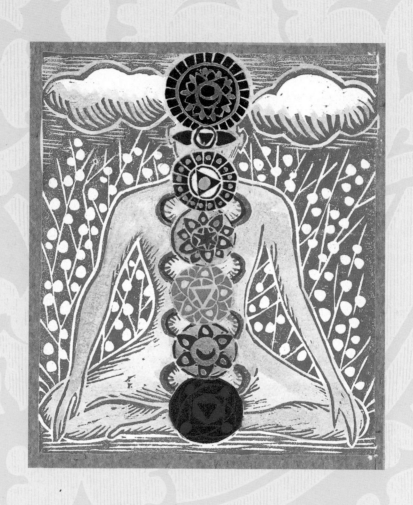

3

WHAT USE ARE CHAKRAS?

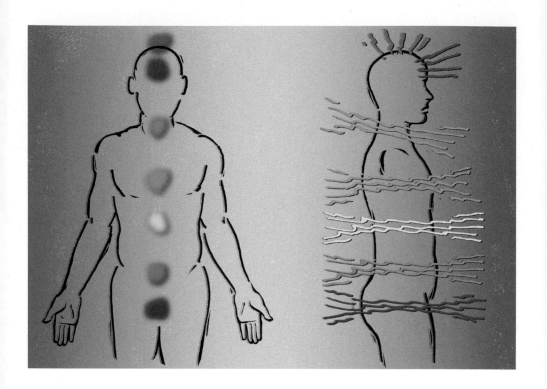

As you read through the chapters on each of the seven main chakras, you may come across character traits and emotional or psychological problems that you recognize within yourself. If this is the case, or if you are focusing on someone else's problems, note down the chakras that best describe their difficulties.

Many physical and emotional health problems require conventional treatment, but complementary remedies can hasten the healing process. Thus, such things as gem therapy, color therapy, massage, reflexology, and spiritual healing can be of use. All of these can be directed toward specific conditions by identifying chakras that need to be cleared, balanced, aligned, mended, or healed.

CHARACTER AND PSYCHOLOGY

Each of the seven main chakras rules a different portion of a person's psychology and character. We all have one or two strong chakras and several weaker ones. We might even have one chakra that is performing very badly indeed. We can strengthen our weaker chakras in various ways:

1. We can work on our psychological health by trying to think, behave, or react in ways that are less harmful to ourselves and to others, but this is practical only if the emotional or psychological problem is fairly mild. Also, it is not always easy to change oneself.
2. Hypnotherapy or emotional freedom technique (a practice in which you stimulate energy meridian points on your body by tapping on them with your fingertips) might be useful.
3. You can ask a healer to channel light and strength into your weaker chakras.
4. You can take advantage of healing techniques such as crystal therapy, color therapy, and aromatherapy. I suggest relevant crystals, colors, and essences for each chakra later in this book.
5. Reflexology, acupuncture, and acupressure all work on the meridian lines, which themselves align to the chakras.
6. Those of you who are into pagan ways may wish to use items that connect to certain chakras on an altar.

PSYCHIC AILMENTS

The chakras are associated with specific body parts and with specific ailments, so healers can work directly on the right chakra for each ailment. For instance, you would work on the sacral and base chakras for bowel problems.

MEDITATION AND PSYCHIC WORK

Your meditations will be more effective if you open your chakras first. The chakras will open easily as soon as you give healing to others or perform any channeling or other kind of spiritual or psychic work. Don't forget to close them again when you have finished.

KUNDALINI

You can raise the power and energy of kundalini, the yogic life force, through the chakra system to connect with the universe, to link with a god or a particular deity, or for specific forms of psychic work. I have included a small chapter on this later in this book.

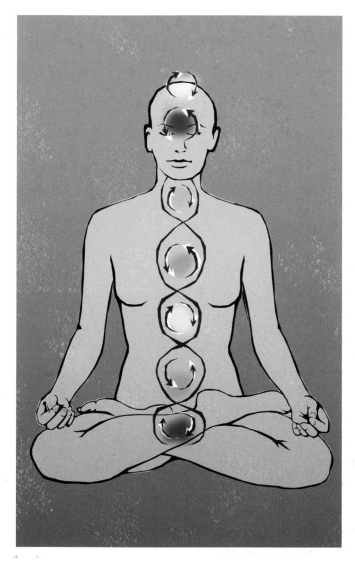

Kundalini

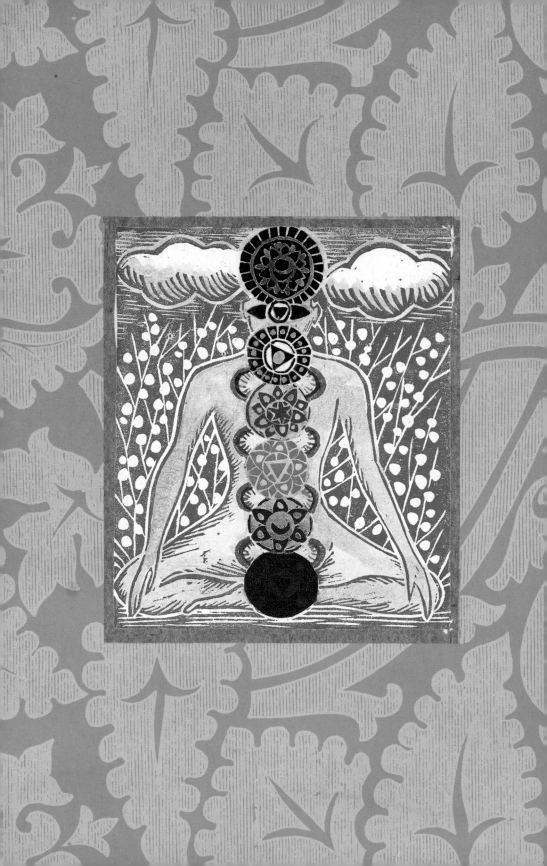

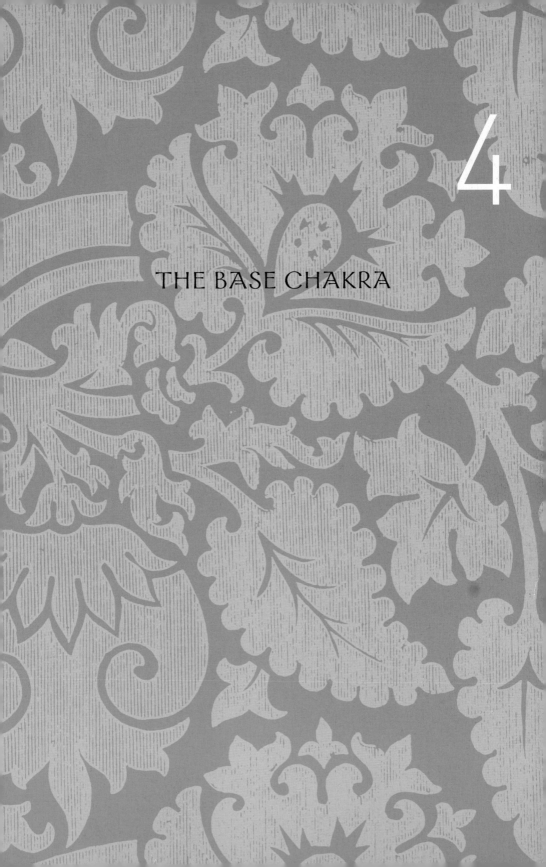

4

THE BASE CHAKRA

Vedic name:	Muladhara
Number:	The first chakra
Other names:	Root chakra, red chakra
Central concept:	Survival, life
Color:	Red
Lotus petals:	Four
Shapes:	Square
Element:	Earth
Planet:	Mars
Zodiac sign:	Scorpio
Health connection:	Legs, base of the body
Balance:	Yang, masculine, positive
Gland:	Adrenal
Sense:	Smell
Mantra:	*Lam*
Music:	Drumming

LOCATION

The base chakra is located at the base of the spine and goes through the body at the bottom of the trunk. Some say that its sphere of influence includes the hips and thighs, while others say that it includes the whole of the legs and feet, linking the body to the earth through the feet.

BASIC PURPOSE

The base chakra symbolizes the drive for survival. It rules such things as the ability to sense danger and to seek safety by taking cover. It also relates to the basis of anything, such as the home from which one ventures out into the world, the mother, one's family history, family honor, the past, the collective unconscious, and even the Earth itself.

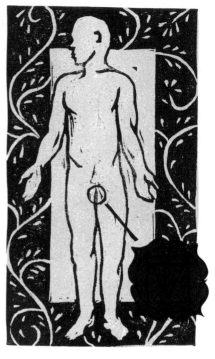

Base Chakra

The realm that is ruled by the base chakra and the one ruled by the sacral chakra, which is the next one up, overlap a little, because both chakras rule parts of the lower trunk, but their attitudes are different from each other. The base chakra is masculine, yang, and active, while the moody sacral chakra is feminine, yin, and more likely to react to situations than to create them. The sexual image of the base chakra is of the act of making love, or even of energetic sex, while the sacral chakra is more involved with the results of making love—for example, pregnancy.

A STRONG BASE CHAKRA

After about six weeks, a baby will begin to look around. It will smile at its mother and it will recognize and respond to the faces and voices of its family members, but those first crucial six weeks are all about survival. An infant needs food, warmth, and protection. It doesn't need an impressive lifestyle or celebrity parents; it needs love and the assurance that it will not be abandoned or uncared for. The base chakra has a similar outlook, as its central concern is self-preservation. There are other topics associated with this chakra, but its main concern is the business of keeping its owner alive and in one piece.

The base chakra is the most down-to-earth and practical of the chakras, because without its influence, we wouldn't have the sense to come in out of the cold or to eat properly. The base chakra gives us our awareness of the world around us, and our place on earth and in society. It rules the need for practical security, including such things as finding a safe area in which to live, obtaining the necessities of life, and making a reasonable lifestyle for ourselves. If danger threatens, the adrenaline associated with this chakra kicks in and stimulates the instinct for fight or flight.

This chakra represents the basis of life and the background that shapes us, and it refers to the kind of family we had and the atmosphere that was around us when we were young. It relates to childhood experiences that affect us many years later.

A friend once told me that when she was a little girl, her father often took up with other women, and, naturally, that made her mother extremely unhappy and angry. Whenever the father sloped off to spend a night with his latest paramour, her mother would take her rage and frustration out on my friend. The sheer terror of coping with a shrieking, out-of-control mother who was lashing out at my friend for some undisclosed and incomprehensible sin was so dreadful that in later life my friend chose to marry a man whose main virtue was that he was unlikely to stray—but that was about his only virtue.

Those with a healthy base chakra are blessed with common sense, a love of the earth, and a love of nature, so folks with a powerful base chakra might be talented gardeners, carpenters, builders, farmers, or civil or mechanical engineers. These individuals are unlikely to be foolish where money and possessions are concerned. They can be assertive, confident, courageous, strong willed, and capable, able to initiate projects and take calculated risks. Individuals with a strong base chakra can find a way of making something that the world will buy, and then go on to build an enterprise and make a great deal of money out of it. They are the workers of the world, and they won't allow others to provide for them or for their families unless absolute disaster occurs, and even then, only until they can get back on their feet. Because of its connection to the need to survive in a financial and practical sense, the base chakra is linked to one's choice of profession.

On a lighter note, this chakra relates to rhythmic music, dance, and the joy of moving to music. The rhythm, movement, and pleasure that we get from playing sports also belong to this chakra. Much the same goes for the pleasure that we get from making love.

Note: I have heard of a good party game that relates to this chakra. Ask a friend to lie down somewhere, and then hold a pendulum over his or her base chakra and allow it to swing back and forth or in a circle. Then ask your friend to think of someone whom he or she is interested in and to think sexy thoughts. Whatever movement the pendulum was making beforehand will change direction now!

Note: Vedic tradition suggests that a person with a strong base chakra will never fear fire, having come into the world knowing that he or she will never be burned in a fire. I guess a person with a strong base chakra would make a good fire-fighter!

Note: Some traditions suggest that the legs and feet belong to a secondary base chakra that might be termed a base-ment chakra, and this chakra relates to energy, love, truth, and unity.

TOO MUCH BASE CHAKRA

People who have too much base chakra can have some good points, and they can earn respect and admiration from others, but they are not easy to live or work with. Some are nice enough, but they are so wrapped up in their work or in making money that they have little time for the niceties of life or for spirituality.

In extreme cases, people with too much base chakra may exhibit troublesome qualities such as addictions to alcohol or sex, and some sufferers display obsessive and compulsive behavior. At the very worst end of the spectrum are people who can't be bothered to understand others or to care about them. They can be selfish and materialistic, greedy, angry, cruel, racist, bigoted, bitchy, and nasty. These problems may be linked to a very low level of self-esteem as well as deep-seated fears, or they can be due to jealousy or an inability to see clearly through a fog of illusion and paranoia.

NOT ENOUGH BASE CHAKRA

Those who have a weak base chakra might live "in their heads," causing them to lack practical, earthy realism. They might be full of self-pity, or they may be weak and frightened. They can be unable to supply themselves with the basic needs in life, and while they have good intentions, they might never quite get around to acting on those intentions. At worst, these individuals are filled with neuroses, anxiety, tension, and terror, with no healthy outlet for their fears.

Note: One simple way to bolster your sense of courage is to wear something red. This color lifts the spirits and increases courage.

BODY AND HEALTH

Needless to say, the ailments associated with the base chakra are those that affect the base of the body. They include cervical erosion, thrush, cystitis, venereal diseases, piles, anal fistulas, prostate problems, testicular problems, sterility, impotence, ejaculation problems, vasectomy, incontinence, vaginal problems, AIDS, constipation, diar-rhea, and much else about the human "plumbing" system that we don't talk about in polite society.

There may also be problems associated with the hips, legs, and feet, including sciatica or troubles with the circulation of blood through the limbs. The base chakra may also be linked to blood pressure levels, arthritis, and some forms of cancer. Along with several other chakras, the base chakra can relate to such "feeding ailments" as anorexia, bulimia, and overeating as part of a mix-up in the survival mechanism and in connection with the pattern of addictive behavior.

This chakra is also said to represent the skeletal system, including the teeth. Its connection to the sense of smell means that the nose is also under its influence.

According to some legends, if a person has a problem with the left hip, leg, or foot, he or she has problems with his or her mother. If the right side is giving the individual problems, the child-father relationship was or is difficult.

Another ancient legend suggests that if you want to heal problems with the base chakra, you should wear pink rather than the traditional red, as pink is gentle and effective rather than angry, hot, and rushed.

SPIRITUAL LINK

The image related to the base chakra is of conception and the start of life, so this chakra symbolizes the starting point of the kundalini journey and the commencement of the search for spirituality. Kundalini is a Hindu concept that involves bringing energy up from the base chakra through the crown and then on up to the heavens or the universe.

Interestingly, despite this being the most basic and earthy chakra, it is where the search for the connection to the divine begins.

Problems might arise for an individual whose base chakra is misaligned because he or she has a particularly rigid attitude to religion, choosing to become part of a world where everything normal is forbidden. This is the realm of self-appointed ayatollahs who enjoy telling others how to live. A healthier form of religious rigidity influenced by the base chakra includes silent orders of monks and nuns. These people give up normal life to focus on serving God, and while we have great respect for them, we all know that this lifestyle is by no means natural, because if we all suddenly took to living in a sequestered convent, the human race wouldn't be able to reproduce itself, and thus it would die off. In one way, belonging to a religious institution is rather like being in the army because those involved don't have to worry about providing for themselves or their families. Their basic needs for food, warmth, clothing, and shelter are met. And so, by this circular route, we are back to square one, which is that the base chakra rules the instinct for survival and basic human needs.

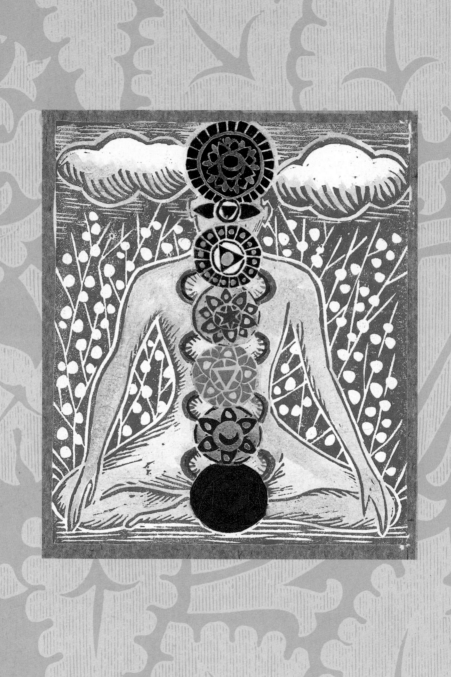

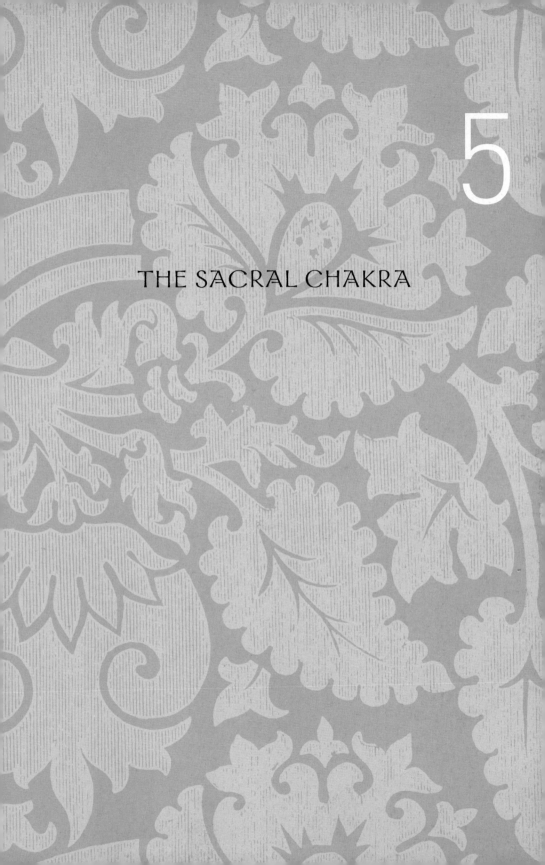

5

THE SACRAL CHAKRA

Vedic name:	Svadhistana
Number:	The second chakra
Other names:	Spleen chakra, orange chakra
Central concept:	Creation, emotions
Color:	Orange
Lotus petals:	Six
Shapes:	Crescent Moon, pyramid
Element:	Water
Planet:	Moon
Zodiac sign:	Cancer
Health connection:	Ovaries, testes
Balance:	Yin, feminine, negative
Gland:	Ovaries, testes
Sense:	Taste
Mantra:	*Vam*
Music:	Strings

LOCATION

The sacral chakra is located in the middle of the abdomen below the navel. It links with the lumbar spine, the sciatic nerve, and the sacral plexus. The Latin name for this chakra is *genitalia*, which matches perfectly with the Vedic connection to the ovaries and testes.

BASIC PURPOSE

The sacral chakra concerns sharing but it also rules independence. The ideal situation is to share with others but not to lean on them or drain them, or, in turn, be drained by others. This chakra rules feelings, emotions, and moods, along with appetites and the desire for sex. However, while base chakra is aggressively masculine and active, the moody sacral chakra is feminine, and the receptive, passive, feminine aspect of this chakra makes it more likely to react to situations than to create them.

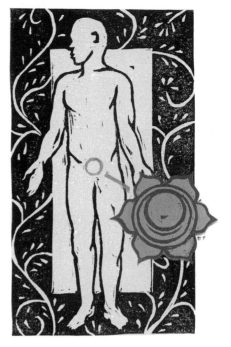

Sacral Chakra

A STRONG SACRAL CHAKRA

The sacral chakra is the largest of all the chakras. It is the seat of the emotions, so it is not surprising that so many people get butterflies in the stomach when they become nervous or excited. Some people get the urge to run to the bathroom before nerve-racking experiences such as performing on the stage.

This chakra connects with the womb, ovaries, and menstrual cycle, so it is associated with mood swings and temperament. The Hindu name for this chakra, Svadhistana, derives from the Sanskrit, as do the ancient Greek and Hebrew names for this chakra, and the word that has come down to us via all these languages is "hysteria"! The ancient Greek name for the womb was "hystera," and it was believed that a woman became hysterical as a direct consequence of a malfunctioning womb! It is true that pain and discomfort in the womb can make a woman short-tempered and depressed, but it is, of course, misguided to attribute all feminine unhappiness to an ailing womb. People of both sexes who suffer back pain, neuralgia, or rheumatism, for example, can be tetchy and bad tempered.

The sacral chakra is linked astrologically to the Moon. Ancient sky watchers considered the Moon restless and temperamental, due to its habit of changing shape, and of seeming to disappear altogether for days on end. The cycles of the Moon have always been linked to the female cycle, and the Moon is metaphorically linked to the "feminine" concepts of intuition, feelings, and hunches. There is a "gut feeling" associated with this chakra.

One very important facet of the sacral chakra is that those who have strong sacral chakras know what's best for themselves. They also know when something or somebody is harmful to them. For instance, someone with a strong sacral chakra will suspect that something is wrong inside his or her body long before anything shows up medically. A strong sacral chakra can also help a person to see or feel that something is wrong with a loved one.

Those who have a strong sacral chakra are able to set boundaries, so they are unlikely to be pushed around, or to be frightened by others or treated as victims. They set sensible rules for their children to follow and they are consistent, so their children know where they stand from one day to the next. These individuals don't make unrealistic sacrifices for others, and they don't become martyrs, so they are pretty content with their environment. They appreciate the good things that they have and they don't complain about what they lack. They focus on what's good in their lives rather than worrying about the things they don't like. They set boundaries for their own behavior. They are pleasant neighbors, good friends, and welcome relatives, who get on with most people and make the best of most situations. Their self-esteem is healthy but not over the top.

This chakra rules sexual attraction as well as the pleasure that one gets from sex. The sacral chakra is associated with creativity; and one form of creativity is the creation of new life; therefore, this chakra rules the desire for children and the desire for a happy family. While we all know that sex can be a solitary pleasure or even a group experience, the reality is that lovemaking is best enjoyed as part of a twosome. It is one of the few things that can be given away to a lover and enjoyed by oneself at the same time. Having a lovely meal is a similar experience because it is so much nicer when shared.

As with the base chakra, the sacral chakra connects a person to the past, the collective unconscious, and his or her family background and roots. The past can influence people in many ways, but someone with a healthy sacral chakra isn't too badly influenced by a bad start in life. This individual develops enough awareness and strength of character to cherry-pick the good things from his or her past and to turn away from the legacy of the bad things. People with a strong sacral chakra can choose to allow the past to influence them or they can choose to forget it. For instance, these individuals may choose to run their homes and family lives in exactly the same way that their parents did, or they may decide to take a very different route. These people may feel that their past experiences, backgrounds, and roots are pretty positive, and they probably feel proud of these things.

Those who have a strong sacral chakra are not in love with money, but they appreciate the freedom that it confers. These folks can succeed in a job or in business by creating goods that people want to buy, and they take pleasure from the creative process of building a business. Their intuitive understanding of other people makes them excellent employers and fine salespeople. They are sociable and somewhat ambitious, although not necessarily money minded. They work well in collective situations where harmony and teamwork are needed. This chakra endows its owners with imagination and intuition, along with a sincere nature and an ability to empathize with others. Needless to say, these people make excellent counselors, healers, nurses, psychic readers, and friends. The motherly nature of this chakra can lead these individuals to create or gather a large family around them or to care for young people on a professional basis.

Vedic tradition suggests that those who have strong sacral chakras come into this world knowing that they will never drown or be harmed by water. I guess someone with a strong sacral chakra would be a successful sailor, swimming pool attendant, or fishing-boat worker!

Note: Tradition also says that every time you are upset by emotional or physical problems related to this chakra, you should take a warm, scented bath.

TOO MUCH SACRAL CHAKRA

When there is too much emphasis on the sacral chakra, cravings and desires can run wild, leading to overeating or addiction to such things as chocolate, alcohol, or prescription drugs. There may be an addiction to appalling relationships. When I worked as an astrologer, I used to come across clients who wanted their lives to be as full of drama and excitement as the soap operas that they watched on television, so they would get involved in relationships that promised this outcome. Their worries inevitably revolved around sex, infidelity, abandonment, and love.

Taken to the extreme, too much sacral chakra can result in jealousy, manipulation, and violent outbursts; excesses of all kinds—even choosing to have more children than the person can cope with—can rule the day.

Someone with an overactive sacral chakra responds well to calming tecniques like meditation, and they also get a lot of benefit from having a massage, aromatherapy reflexology, or a head massage. The sacral chakra is attuned to water, so a swim in a warm pool or relaxation in a spa bath also helps to lower the tension level.

NOT ENOUGH SACRAL CHAKRA

In some individuals in which there is not enough sacral chakra, there is a kind of choice going on; it's not so much a personality problem as a lifestyle choice that leads the person away from loving or sexual relationships. For example, there are some who put their energies into work instead of family life, and while this is not necessarily a bad thing, it can make for a rather one-sided lifestyle. We have all read about tycoons who spend so much time at work that either they don't have partners, or, if they do marry, sooner or later their partners wander off and find someone who's actually around and who shows some interest in them. Some people with a weak sacral chakra relate well to animals, which shows they have loving natures, but this love is not directed at other human beings. In severe cases, those with a very weak sacral chakra are timid, withdrawn, and nervous. They may be frightened of getting involved with others because they lack romance or real emotion. They find it hard to understand or empathize with other people. They may become victims or martyrs when in relationships.

Sometimes people with a weak sacral chakra can be so busy doing things for others that they put their own needs last, so that they end up feeling as though they have lost themselves.

BODY AND HEALTH

The sacral chakra rules the organs of procreation: the uterus, ovaries, and fallopian tubes in women, and the testes in men. Problems related to fertility come under this chakra. Many ailments associated with the sacral chakra are similar to those of the base chakra, so we might find problems related to the womb, ovaries, and fallopian tubes, as well as the bowels. The sacral chakra also rules impotence, prostate problems, and frigidity, and such things as fibroids and ovarian cysts. This area rules lower-back pain, slipped discs, sciatica, and pain in the long muscles of the lower back, along with movement and walking affected by lower-back conditions.

Some say that this chakra rules the organs of sex and fertility only in women, but not in men. They say that the sacral chakra rules the spleen in men. As in so many esoteric fields, there are differences of opinions.

The sacral chakra rules nourishment, so it relates to eating problems, including overeating, anorexia, and bulimia. Allergic conditions such as migraine and candida albicans can be found in the area governed by the sacral chakra, as can be asthma and eczema. There is also a link between the sacral chakra and depression and dissatisfaction with life.

SPIRITUAL LINK

Whereas the base chakra rules the moment of conception, the sacral chakra represents the early stages of growth. The sacral chakra rules the time when a person is searching for spirituality but doesn't yet know which direction to take. This chakra is linked with feelings and intuition, so it will trigger unsettled feelings that warn us when something is wrong. On a less dramatic level, the sacral chakra governs those times when an individual thinks of someone, only to have that person to contact the individual later that day.

Some psychics say that this is by far the largest chakra, so if you need to be intuitive or psychic and don't have the time to go through the process of opening and closing all the chakras, open just this one. Always remember to close the chakra afterward, though.

EXAMPLE OF AN INDIVIDUAL WITH A STRONG SACRAL CHAKRA

My friend Gerry has a strong sacral chakra, so, depending upon your point of view, Gerry could be considered to be either a sucker or a kind and thoughtful person. As an artist, writer, broadcaster, and entertainer, Gerry doesn't have a steady income, but despite this, his friends and family expect him to keep them in style and to run around after them. They frequently expect him to put his own life on hold for their benefit. Each of them thinks he or she has every right to his time, money, and energy. Some of them don't realize that there are several people draining him. Others know this but don't care. Gerry could try to improve things by meditating on his condition and by asking his spiritual guides to strengthen his sacral chakra, or he could go to an energy healer for healing that is directed into his sacral chakra. This might make him more able to recognize what is reasonable or unreasonable and thus save him much unnecessary trouble.

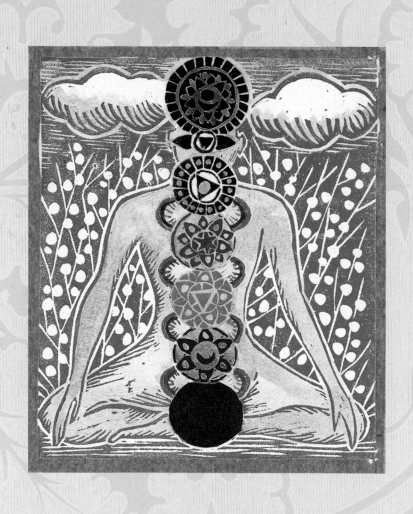

6

THE SOLAR PLEXUS CHAKRA

Vedic name:	Manipura
Number:	The third chakra
Other names:	Yellow chakra, naval chakra
Central concept:	Energy, control, belief
Color:	Yellow
Lotus petals:	Ten
Shapes:	Circle
Element:	Fire
Planet:	Sun
Zodiac sign:	Leo
Health connection:	Digestion
Balance:	Yang, masculine, positive
Gland:	Pancreas, endocrine
Sense:	Sight
Mantra:	*Ram*
Music:	Reeds, horns

LOCATION

The solar plexus chakra is located just above the navel.

BASIC PURPOSE

The solar plexus chakra is associated with the ability to achieve one's aims and ambitions; thus, it is linked to courage and self-confidence. It rules curiosity, the desire to acquire knowledge, and the desire to obtain the right kind of experience. Issues surrounding control and freedom can be found associated with this chakra. On the one hand, this symbolizes the self-control and the latitude that a person allows himself or herself; on the other hand, it can relate to the ability to direct and control others.

A successful person has a definite purpose in life and a fair chance of achieving his or her aims. Combine this with comfortable relationships, good friendships, good health, an active mind, interesting pastimes, and the ability to have a good laugh from time to time, and we have the definition of a perfectly happy person. This chakra rules the *prana*, or life force, and its allied concept of happiness. Naturally, the best relationship is the one we have with ourselves, so this chakra is about self-acceptance and self-worth, rather than self-consciousness or being one's own worst critic.

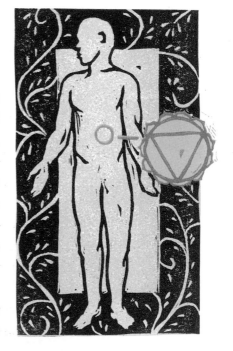

Solar Plexus Chakra

A STRONG SOLAR PLEXUS CHAKRA

When the sunny solar plexus chakra is working properly, it allows an individual to be happy and successful. It endows the individual with energy, willpower, and get-up-and-go. These lucky people have the confidence and courage to tackle new projects and the ability to see them through. They are alert and open to new initiatives and ideas, and they have the endurance to finish what they start.

These folks know their own strengths; they don't get into fights and arguments for the sake of it, but they can stand up for themselves when necessary. They have leadership qualities but they are neither domineering nor aggressive. They can choose to make sacrifices for loved ones on occasion, but they won't allow themselves to become martyrs or victims.

The connection between the solar plexus chakra and the ability to study makes these folks good students and good teachers. The current emphasis on data and information suits these individuals, because these people can absorb any amount of data. They become like walking encyclopedias, but they need to guard against becoming know-it-alls or bores.

Money is important to these individuals, but seeing themselves as successful and commanding the respect and admiration of others are stronger motivators. Whether their area of operation is business or whether their ambitions point them in other directions, they will be eager to excel at something. Knowledge can be seen as power, and at the least, it can prevent others from walking all over them when it comes to negotiating. Someone with a fully functioning solar plexus chakra will make sure he or she is equipped with all the necessary information before walking into a difficult situation. These people are grounded, secure, and comfortable within the arenas in which they operate. They are decisive, capable, and intelligent, with a healthy sense of self-worth and a very good sense of humor. They don't go through life fearing illness or death, and they seldom get sick.

The downside, even when this chakra is relatively well balanced, is that these individuals can make a mess of relationships. Loving relationships are not about winning, or even about being the most exciting, richest, and most charismatic person around. They are about love and respect for a partner, along with give-and-take. These workaholic, persistent, pernickety, successful individuals may shine in the wider world, but they don't always make a success of relationships.

Note: An ancient traditional source suggests that these people are never likely to be in danger from fire, and they don't fear fire.

TOO MUCH SOLAR PLEXUS CHAKRA

Individuals with too much solar plexus chakra can be cold, logical, and analytical and may use logical arguments to demolish the opinions of others. They make admirable computer programmers or analysts, because a computer doesn't have emotions, of course. They abuse power, either by being argumentative, loud, and physical or by being cold and calculating.

At the very worst end of the spectrum, those who have an overabundance of solar plexus chakra energy are arrogant, angry, and irritable. They may be domineering or power hungry. They can be hurtful and sarcastic, and they may not hold back from attacking others physically either. Alternatively, they can be fussy perfectionists who like to impose their obsessive standards on others, while allowing themselves plenty of leeway. They can be witty and amusing at times, but it is unpleasant to be around them for too long. They fear being alone and therefore find ways of binding others to them.

NOT ENOUGH SOLAR PLEXUS CHAKRA

Some people fall behind in the career success race due to increasing age or because they spend so much time at home with small children. Sometimes staying at home turns the mind to mush, so if these folk want to improve the action of their solar plexus chakras, they should take classes, learn a sport, or take dancing lessons. They should do puzzles, jigsaws, and crosswords, read books, and, if possible, get out and interact with others. This chakra is about curiosity, wit, humor, and awareness, so anything that increases the mental faculties will build up a weak solar plexus chakra.

In the worst cases, these individuals can be too flexible for their own good. They are people pleasers who lack the courage to negotiate for their own rights and requirements. They lack the confidence, intelligence, energy, and luck that would help them to succeed with a project. A lethal cocktail of poor self-esteem, fear of risk, and shortage of verve hold these folks back. They attract the attention of bullies, and they can be pessimists and losers. They might be apathetic and inert, they may lack intelligence, and they certainly lack passion. These individuals find it hard to make decisions, so they can abruptly make wrong choices, sometimes out of fear or even in a fit of pique. They are too self-effacing. Some can be successful on a superficial level, but they gain advantage by being slippery and treacherous, and they may delude themselves about their worth and their abilities.

BODY AND HEALTH

Can you stomach it? Well, if you can't, chances are that your solar plexus chakra is in trouble. This may be a temporary problem such as a stomach upset. The solar plexus chakra rules the digestive organs, stomach, liver, pancreas, and gall bladder. Individuals with a misaligned solar plexus chakra have difficulty converting food into energy, perhaps due to stomach ulcers, liver problems, gallstones, diabetes, or hypoglycemia. An individual affected in this way may often feel fatigued or may gain or lose too much weight.

In some countries, there are parasites that enter the body through the skin or by other means, living in their host until they have completed part of their breeding or growing cycle. Two ailments that result from this type of infection are malaria and schistosomiasis, and they are associated with this chakra. The solar plexus chakra rules the skin and the sense of sight, so it is allied to the eyes.

SPIRITUAL LINK

Individuals who have strong solar plexus chakras know their own strength and tend to use it for the benefit of others. They don't pull others down or compete with them, because this doesn't give them pleasure. On the contrary, they obtain pleasure by helping others reach their potential. The happiness, wit, and humor of people with strong solar plexus chakras can be used to bring fun and joy to others. These individuals make excellent parents, and some of them choose to look after other people's children, and to help youngsters develop skills and confidence. These individuals can encourage others to gain vision and clarity and make the best of themselves. Such people can be the bridge between the day-to-day world of material success, on the one hand, and the need to pray and thank the Almighty for his help, on the other.

Note: One ancient tradition suggests that people with a strong solar plexus chakra have the ability to travel astrally. If you want to try this, start by relaxing on your bed, and then, as you start to become sleepy, imagine yourself leaving your body, rising, and traveling away for a while. You should be able to get back into your body again, but it can be somewhat unnerving if you find it difficult to climb back in!

EXAMPLE OF AN INDIVIDUAL WITH A STRONG SOLAR PLEXUS CHAKRA

Andrew has a strong solar plexus, which gives him amazing belief in himself, and this helps to make him a worldly success story. He runs a business that spans the world, and he spends his life in airplanes, dropping down from a great height into one head office after another to check on the figures and to give his opinion. He hires the best people for his company and quickly gets rid of those who don't come up to scratch. He has spent many years looking for the right partner, and now he seems to have found one. Interestingly, his partner is a Capricorn—a sign that is known for making advantageous marriages and for a love of trendy, expensive possessions and high status.

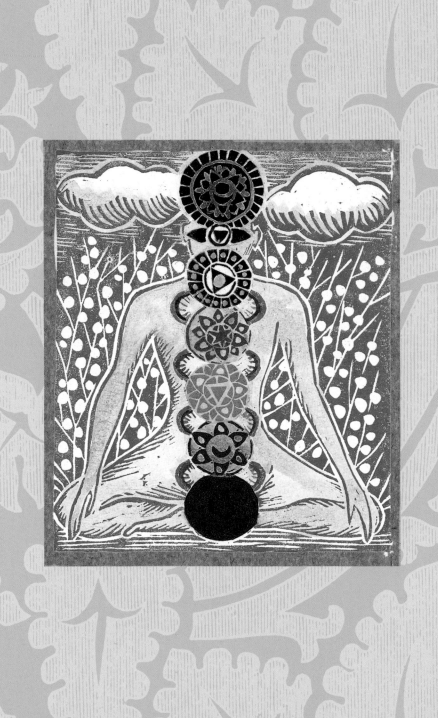

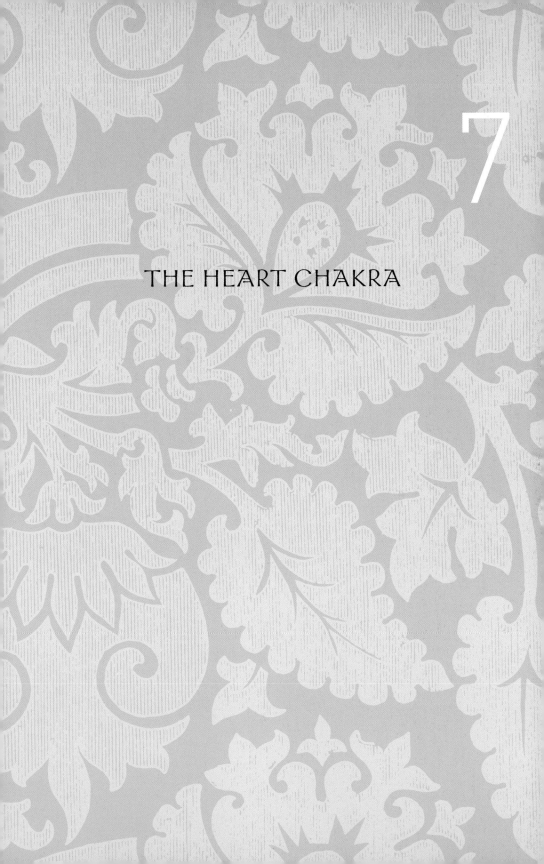

7

THE HEART CHAKRA

Vedic name:	Anahata
Number:	The fourth chakra
Other names:	Green chakra
Central concept:	Love, relating, respect, creativity
Color:	Green
Lotus petals:	Twelve
Shapes:	Cross
Element:	Air
Planet:	Venus
Zodiac sign:	Libra
Health connection:	Heart, lungs, upper digestive tract
Balance:	Yin, feminine, negative
Gland:	Thymus
Sense:	Touch
Mantra:	*Yam*
Music:	Flute, woodwinds

LOCATION

Unsurprisingly, the heart chakra is based in the center of the chest in the area of the heart. It is associated with the heart, lungs, thorax, upper digestive tract, and ribs.

BASIC PURPOSE

The heart chakra is concerned with love and also with the ability to relate to others. It is also associated with the ability to love and respect ourselves, to be creative, and to be wise. This chakra is the gateway between the humanity-oriented lower chakras and the more divinely oriented upper chakras. The heart chakra is concerned with emotional security and with loving comfort. It seeks to form a balance between the need for love and the need for spiritual excellence, so it rules selflessness, compassion, devotion, and a sensible measure of sacrifice on behalf of others. The heart chakra concerns physical and emotional healing, but also creativity, artistry, music, and crafts. In a way, it is also connected to the ideas of those things that offer us fun, amusement, and uplift, in addition to relaxation, rest, and recovery.

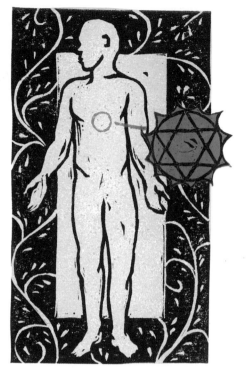

Heart Chakra

A STRONG HEART CHAKRA

Those with strong heart chakras are loving and unselfish, but they don't allow themselves to become martyrs or to be manipulated by others. These people don't flee from emotional commitment, because they are happy to love others, but they like to be loved in return. They don't need to play games. They forgive themselves when they do something wrong, and they understand and forgive others. Those with strong heart chakras neither hoard money nor spend it foolishly, and they are neither stingy nor extravagant. They are balanced in every aspect of their lives. Those who have a strong heart chakra are reasonable to live with, work alongside, and be around because they have a healthy dose of self-respect and they also gain the respect of others. Some of those with a strong heart chakra make a calculated decision to give up the chance of fun and freedom in order to take care of sick relatives, while others might even take up vocations in religious orders. Many choose to work with the needy.

Brian Cartwright is a real-life example of a person with a strong heart chakra. He gave up a well-paid job that he hated so that he could teach individuals with physical disabilities how to fix cars. He loved seeing his students develop their new skills and gain confidence, and it gave him a real thrill when the organization that he worked for managed to find jobs for his students. Brian didn't earn much money, but it didn't matter because his wife was a highflyer with a good salary. They had two sons who loved and respected both parents, so everyone was happy—great heart chakras all around in that family!

One aspect of the heart chakra is the ability to cope when times are bad, which means that these individuals can handle loss, separation, bereavement, and heartache with a degree of equilibrium. People with strong heart chakras are not cold or unemotional, but they don't fall into a heap of self-pity or dejection when things go wrong. They have a measure of spiritual acceptance, and they know that even bad times are necessary for growth and understanding. These folks hope for the best, and they trust others unless they find a good reason not to.

People with strong heart chakras often choose careers that involve working with people. They work in the public sector or in jobs that require teamwork and that help people in some way. They work with children, the elderly, the weak, individuals with disabilities, or those who need advice. If they don't need money, they often take up voluntary work.

In a person with a strong heart chakra, there is a measure of self-acceptance and self-knowledge, so this person knows that, while he or she may not be perfect, he or she is pretty much all right.

TOO MUCH HEART CHAKRA

Individuals with too much heart chakra can put the needs of others above their own to a ridiculous extent, perhaps by choosing a partner who is very needy or who needs to be rescued. The partner might have a weakness for alcohol, drugs, gambling, or some other destructive habit. Misplaced loyalty is common in people with an overabundance of heart chakra.

At the worst end of the spectrum, people with too much heart chakra can be manipulative and possessive or fond of making emotional scenes. Their love is conditional because it is doled out only when the other person does what they want, and they withhold love just when the other person most needs it. They can make a partner's or child's life a complete misery. Sometimes the person is self-centered, possessive, and jealous, or power hungry, bitter, and prone to hatred. This individual finds it impossible to forgive.

NOT ENOUGH HEART CHAKRA

Just as an angry and confrontational person can drive others away, so can a whining, self-pitying, dependent one. Both behaviors are a form of manipulation. As we have seen, those with too much heart chakra can give too much of themselves to others; similarly, so can individuals with not enough heart chakra, because this behavior can represent two sides of the same coin. Some people give far too much of themselves in the vain hope of obtaining or maintaining the approval of others.

In many ways, the heart chakra is about courage. All situations that involve relating to others, whether at home, at work, or elsewhere, require courage, common sense, and the ability to set limits. Thus, those who lack heart chakra energy may allow others to walk all over them. Alternatively, they might feel unlovable or unworthy of love. Such individuals might be stuck in a rut and lack the courage or energy to move out of it. Other problems might arise due to fear of the future. People without enough heart chakra might be paralyzed by envy or may feel unattractive, immobile, and helpless to effect change in their lives.

Interestingly, an individual with an insufficiency of heart chakra may be perfectly happy, but just not interested in romantic love or in relationships at all. He or she may get fulfillment in life through other routes—perhaps by creating a great garden or great art, by looking after pets, or through an absorbing job or hobby.

BODY AND HEALTH

Naturally, the heart is ruled by this chakra, but the heart chakra also rules the circulation, lungs, and rib cage. The heart chakra is associated with such ailments as asthma, allergies, and pneumonia, and it is also associated with problems in the upper spine and shoulders. The heart chakra is metaphorically linked to the air element, so it rules breathing difficulties. Those with a powerful heart chakra might cough or find it hard to breathe when they are upset or excited. This chakra also rules the immune system; therefore, it is associated with AIDS, type 1 diabetes, cell growth, and blood pressure. The heart chakra is also associated with the thymus and growth hormones, and it rules the shoulders, arms, and breasts.

SPIRITUAL LINK

Tradition says that the heart chakra is associated with out-of-body experiences and with flying to the astral universe. It also rules spiritual knowledge, so those who have a healthy heart chakra make wonderful counselors, healers, doctors, psychologists, and therapists. Some spiritual healers feel this chakra opening when they start to work.

Those who have a strong heart chakra can make excellent salespeople. They like and understand people, so they know instinctively how to make customers feel comfortable. This chakra can denote putting one's heart into some things like charitable work and social work that are for the benefit of others.

EXAMPLES OF INDIVIDUALS WITH STRONG HEART CHAKRAS

In 1985, Bob Geldof went from scruffy pop singer to prime mover against suffering in Africa, and he has worked in the field ever since. Not only did he raise his own three children after the death of their mother, Paula Yates, but he also took care of her child by another man. Bob's big heart and his tremendous heart chakra are warm and wonderful.

Another example of an individual with a strong heart chakra begins with a woman's struggle for balance, and with a daughter who used her mother's love and guilt to get her own way at every turn.

Joanne brought her daughter along for a reading with me. Joanne was a nice-looking woman, but her daughter, Tracy, was an overweight girl who spent her days slumped in front of the television and eating. Joanne wanted something better for her daughter, but she also had an agenda of her own. After a difficult marriage, an even more difficult divorce, and time spent getting back on her feet financially, Joanne was ready to get out and socialize. Joanne figured that the presence of overweight, underperforming daughter as a fixture in the middle of her living room wouldn't help her achieve her social ambitions and would definitely put the block on any romantic ambitions that Joanne might harbor.

Tracy was well aware of her mother's desire for a life of her own, so she did all she could to resist this call to change, but Joanne's primordial urge to start a new life was forcing her to fight Tracy's tyranny of inertia and to create a better balance in her own life and in her own heart chakra.

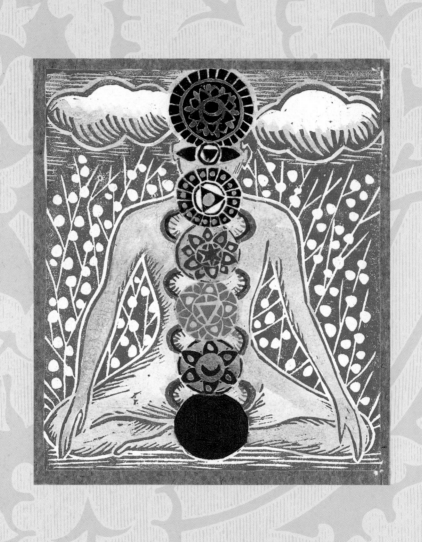

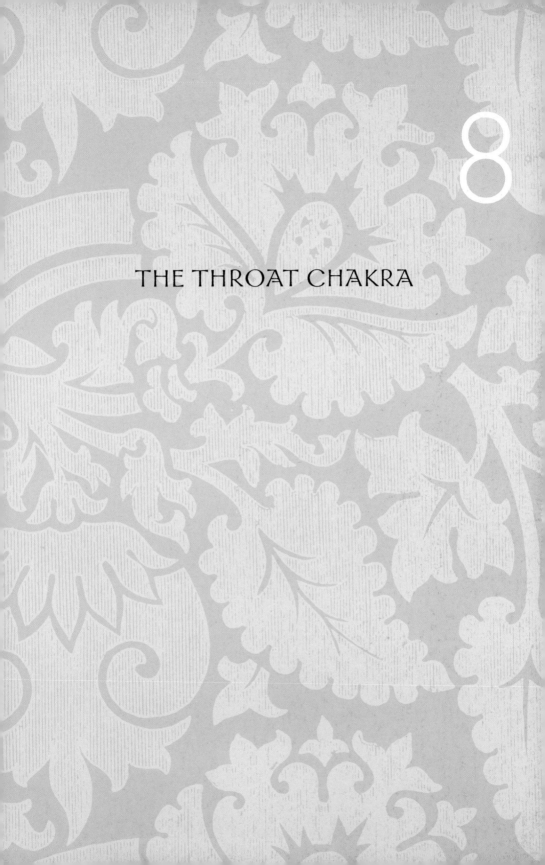

8

THE THROAT CHAKRA

Vedic name:	Vishuddha
Number:	The fifth chakra
Other names:	Light blue chakra
Central concept:	Communication
Color:	Sky blue
Lotus petals:	Sixteen
Shapes:	Cup
Element:	Air/Ether
Planet:	Mercury
Zodiac sign:	Virgo
Health connection:	Throat
Balance:	Yang, masculine, positive
Gland:	Thyroid, parathyroid
Sense:	Hearing
Facial area:	Throat
Mantra:	*Ham*
Music:	Singing

LOCATION

The throat chakra runs through the neck from the lower part of the throat to the lower part of the cervical spine, more or less where it joins the shoulders. The throat chakra rules the thyroid and parathyroid, ears, mouth, and lower face. It also concerns the neck, the top of the shoulders, and the upper spine, along with the upper areas of the bronchial system. It is associated with speech and hearing.

BASIC PURPOSE

The throat chakra rules communication and language. Apart from the obvious matter of being able to get a point across and argue a case, this chakra also symbolizes communication in the form of writing, poetry, music, and art. A less obvious form of communication is the ability to listen and to really hear what others are saying.

In a practical sense, the throat chakra controls growth and the development of the growth glands and growth hormones. In a metaphorical sense, it is also associated with the concept of growth of character through experience. Part of being an adult is the ability to take personal responsibility, so this is another attribute of a healthy throat chakra. On a more mundane level, which is nevertheless extremely important, it rules the ability to work and earn money.

Note: Tradition says this chakra is associated with the sixteen vowels in the Sanskrit language.

A STRONG THROAT CHAKRA

The throat chakra is associated with logic, reason, and common sense. People with strong throat chakras are loyal, calm, tactful, and trustworthy. They take responsibility for their own

Throat Chakra

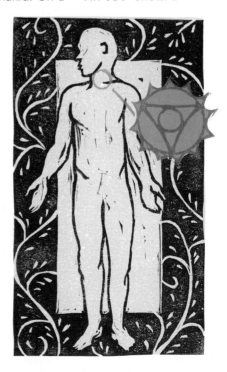

67

actions and don't blame others for their own shortcomings; nor do they blame others when things go wrong. They exude authority. These people can see through lies and manipulation, their instincts are good, and because they enjoy argument and debate, they may be drawn to careers in legal work or politics. They take personal responsibility for their decisions, set realistic goals, and get things done. They succeed in the material world and they live fulfilling lives. However, when things don't work out as they had planned, they are able to accept what cannot be. They are realistic.

Those who have an abundant and healthy throat chakra are independent, so they rarely lean on others. They have an instinctive knowledge, however, that the universe or some higher power exists, so when they need help, they know that they can pray for it and receive it. There is an unconscious spiritual attitude to everything they do, so they are honest, decent, and charitable toward others.

These people can be persuasive, so they negotiate well and can be excellent salespeople. They can cope with accounting, budget, and treasury work, business communications, and making deals that work for all the parties concerned. A strong throat chakra encourages individuals to stretch themselves, to accept challenges, and to aim high. These people can envisage the future that they want: they can see where they want to be, and they can work backward from that point to create a strategy for achieving their aims. They are good at long-term planning, but they may be less able to deal with details than others are.

Note: Some traditions say that the back part of this chakra (the back of the neck) relates to one's profession and one's place in society, while the front area concerns communication and hearing.

TOO MUCH THROAT CHAKRA

Those who have too much throat chakra express their opinions easily but don't stop and listen to what others have to say. They may be prejudiced, rigid, and opinionated. They can't empathize with those who are different from them or whose ideas and opinions are not like theirs.

At the worst end of the spectrum, these people can be intolerant. They blame others, and they refuse to take personal responsibility for things that go wrong. They may be talkative, arrogant, self-righteous, spiteful, and boring. They never express sympathy or feel empathy for others. At heart, these loud, bullying people are actually cowards who don't have the courage of their convictions.

They avoid work, or cherry-pick the nice jobs and leave the boring or dirty jobs for others to do. They take credit for the ideas and achievements of others. At heart, they are jealous of others.

Some people talk at the top of their voices to intimidate people, while others like to exert control by talking so quietly that their "audience" must focus fully on them while they are speaking. This is the kind of technique used by Marlon

Brando when he was acting in the film *The Godfather*. Both techniques are indicative of an aggressive and overused throat chakra.

NOT ENOUGH THROAT CHAKRA

Individuals who are lacking in throat chakra are their own worst enemies, because they don't stand up for themselves or speak up when they feel an injustice. Sometimes they attract bullies into their lives, in the mistaken belief that the bully is a strong person who will protect them. Some characters with a weak throat chakra may lie to save the feelings of others or to protect themselves from someone else's anger. They are dishonest with themselves, but they may feel that is the only way they can cope. They may live with impossible situations because they are afraid to speak up, or walk out of a bad situation and face the uncertainty of a new one. Some accept too much blame and shame for things that are beyond their control.

At worst they whine, they are pessimists, and they blame others for everything. They can be crafty or they may use manipulation to get their own way. They look backward and wallow in memories of the past. These individuals harbor grudges.

BODY AND HEALTH

Naturally, the throat chakra is associated with the throat, but it is also connected to the respiratory system and the vocal cords. This chakra rules colds, flu, coughs, asthma, allergies, ulcers, sore throats, tonsillitis, laryngitis, and the like. It rules the jaw, the teeth, and the start of the digestive system, which includes swallowing, reflux, and hiatal hernias. It can be associated with eating disorders such as anorexia and bulimia. It also rules the thyroid and parathyroid glands, so it can relate to growth and development through its connection with growth hormones.

The throat chakra is associated with the ears, so it is connected to deafness and the organs of balance. When this chakra needs healing, chanting can help, as can listening to music, dancing, and moving rhythmically.

In women, the throat chakra is linked to the menstrual cycle, PMS, menopause, mood swings, night sweats, fevers, and itches.

SPIRITUAL LINK

It is the spiritual aspect of this chakra that is the most important, because this chakra symbolizes the crossing point between the mundane world and the realm of Spirit. The traditional task for the throat chakra is purification, because it acts as a filter that traps issues that come up from the earthly chakras before they can be drawn up into the heavenly chakras that lie above. Some people think that materialism and unpleasant emotions like jealousy can prevent us from tapping into deities and the heavenly realms. They believe that this chakra acts as a filter that keeps these unpleasant desires and emotions away from these realms.

This chakra helps people to pray, chant, and access the universe. We can help the throat chakra to do its work by using such techniques as drumming, humming, chanting mantras, singing hymns or sacred songs, or praying. This chakra allows people to pray for what they need and to tune in to their inner voices.

Specifically, this chakra rules clairaudience, so a well-aligned throat chakra is an essential aid to those who have the rare gift of being able to hear Spirit.

EXAMPLES OF INDIVIDUALS WITH STRONG THROAT CHAKRAS

Gwendolyn had a strong throat chakra. She expressed herself easily and had a wonderful speaking voice. If others had the temerity to disagree with or criticize her, she didn't hesitate to straighten them out. Gwendolyn was never at a loss for words in any situation. On a positive note, she learned early in childhood that nobody was going to give her a free ride in life—least of all her weak parents. When she realized that the school that she attended was worthless, she took herself off to a better one without even bothering to tell her parents. Gwendolyn ended up owning and running a highly successful printing business, and after several failed relationships she even ended up in a happy marriage.

George, another individual with a strong throat chakra, came from a poor background. His father worked for a railroad and his mother never worked at all because she pretended to be sick during the early part of his childhood. Then she "got religion" and became a pillar of her local church and a busybody in the local branch of the Salvation Army.

George knew that he wasn't a natural academic, so when he came out of the air force after World War II, he took advantage of the free training programs that were offered to ex-servicemen and became an electrician. He went into industry and then into management and eventually became a top civil service executive in the Atomic Energy Commission.

There is no doubt that George was a tough guy and a bully, but he looked after his family well, and they never wanted for anything. Who but someone with such a strong sense of his own wonderfulness could make a success after such a mundane start in life?

Note: Interestingly, although he never smoked a cigarette in his life, George eventually died of throat cancer.

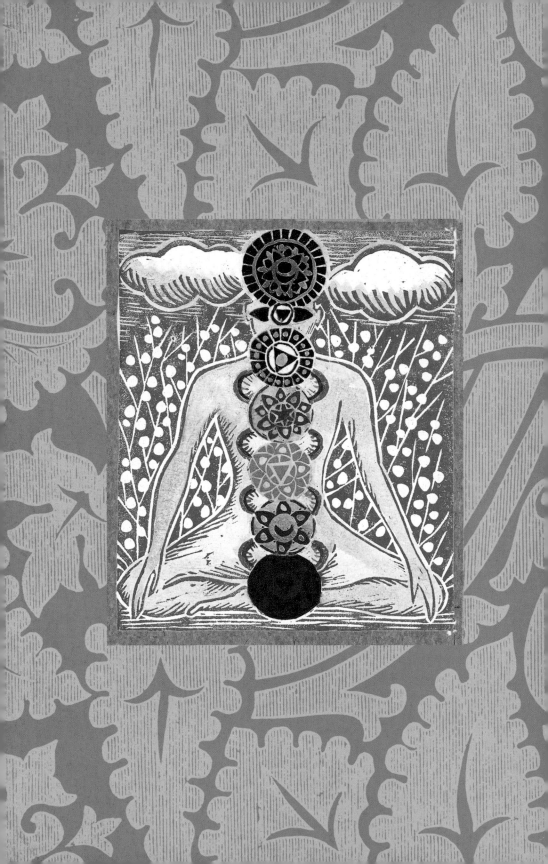

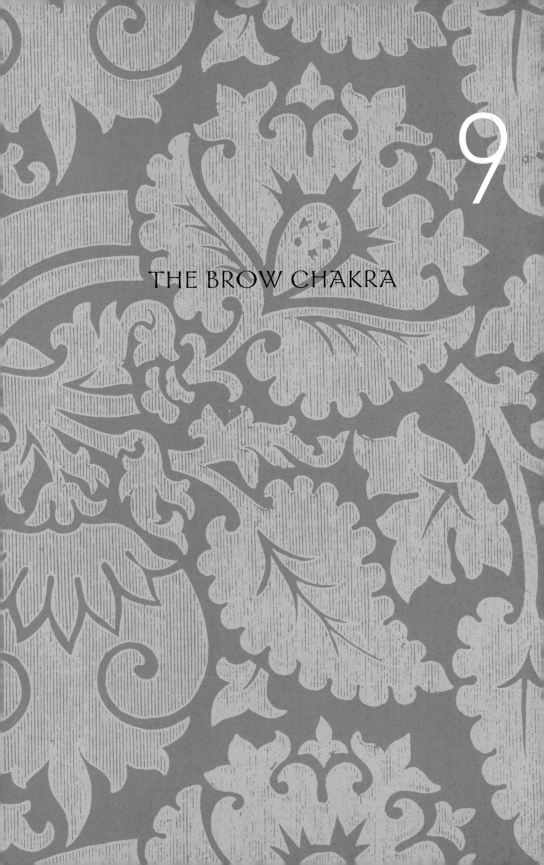

9

THE BROW CHAKRA

Vedic name:	Ajna
Number:	The sixth chakra
Other names:	Third eye chakra, frontal chakra, indigo chakra
Central concept:	Knowledge, clarity
Color:	Indigo blue
Lotus petals:	A circle with a petal on each side
Shapes:	Star of David
Element:	Light
Planet:	Jupiter
Zodiac sign:	Pisces
Health connection:	Head
Balance:	Yang, masculine, positive
Gland:	Pineal/Pituitary
Sense:	Sight
Facial area:	Eyes, skull
Mantra:	*Aum*
Music:	Sacred songs and music

LOCATION

The brow chakra is often called the third eye. Some say that it is located between the eyes, while others believe that it sits in the center of the forehead. Some sources say it rules the pineal gland, and others say it rules the pituitary gland.

BASIC PURPOSE

The brow chakra is concerned with the connection to the spirit world, so it rules such things as extrasensory perception and the ability to contact or receive messages from Spirit. It is an essential part of channeling and spiritual healing.

On a mundane level, it rules self-knowledge and being able to take responsibility for one's own actions.

A STRONG BROW CHAKRA

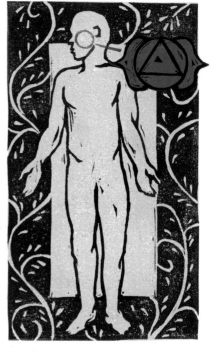

Brow Chakra

The brow chakra is concerned with vision, in the sense of receiving and being able to interpret clairvoyant visions and the information that comes in the form of dreams or symbols. This chakra rules everything connected to second sight and spirit messages. The brow chakra opens very quickly. If you try your hand at tarot readings, it will open without any great effort, and if you watch tarot readers working, you will often see them absentmindedly rubbing their foreheads while doing so. This chakra is especially useful in visualization, in meditation, and for those who have the gift of seeing auras. It is linked to remote viewing and intuition. It allows the individual to see through other people and to pick up on their real motives.

This sector rules thought, ideas, and inspiration, particularly ideas that one can actually bring to life, for example, writing a play and then seeing it performed on the stage. There is a symbolic idea associated with the brow chakra that connects to routes, roadways, and pathways, so someone with a strong brow chakra can find a way through a dilemma or can locate a route or pathway that leads from one situation to another.

The brow chakra is associated with memory, but it doesn't cling to the past or harbor bitterness about it, because it rules the ability to learn from past hurts and to move on from them, even when memories of the events themselves still linger. In practical terms, a strong brow chakra endows people with decency, faithfulness, sympathy for others, clear sight, idealism, and integrity. It brings a reverence for all life and a responsible attitude to everything. Those who have strong brow chakras can take responsibility for themselves and for their own actions, and can also take care of those who need their strength.

Individuals with strong brow chakras should pursue careers that have long-term goals, such as jobs in local government, the insurance industry, pensions, civil engineering, or town planning. These people are visionaries, so having the courage to visualize something and make it happen should suit them. If they take on the responsibility for a fund-raising event, for example, they will soon find the right people to help them.

Note: The Sanskrit word "*ajna*" means "to command"; in this case, it means to take command of one's own life and to bring ideas and concepts to fruition in a carefully controlled manner. If you have a healthy brow chakra, you display leadership skills and you earn the respect of others.

Note: Tradition links this chakra to the relationship with the mother and to a person's feelings about his or her mother.

TOO MUCH BROW CHAKRA

Too much brow chakra is a sign of those who are badly behaved, but who ignore or excuse their own bad behavior, while at the same time judging others and finding them wanting. These individuals are obstinate, and their minds are stuck in a rut. They hide from the truth and can be bossy, domineering, insensitive, and full of superiority. They display little concern for others and have even less contact with reality. They are totally absorbed in their own needs and desires.

A rather odd product of an overpowering brow chakra is the spiritual bore. These individuals discover the world of mediums, ESP, ghosts, and so forth, and they become so immersed in it that they lose touch with reality and forget to use their common sense. Like all bores, they only have one topic of conversation, and they lack balance.

In the worst of cases, their strong opinions can lead them to be racist or xenophobic.

NOT ENOUGH BROW CHAKRA

Individuals without enough brow chakra lack self-confidence and are short on self-esteem. They are sensitive and easily hurt, and they suffer from feelings of inadequacy. They can buy into and actually believe the opinions of those who enjoy putting them down. They overanalyze or overrationalize situations, and they find it hard to move on after a put-down. Not unexpectedly, these features might be a legacy of a poor childhood or the result of a past-life situation.

These people are intuitive but unfocused, so they don't achieve much and never manage to build up their self-confidence. They sacrifice too much to others. They may put themselves last to keep the peace or because they don't know how to stand up for themselves. There is a fine line between admiration and envy, and those with a poor brow chakra find themselves crossing it.

Sometimes circumstances that are beyond their control lead to isolation and loneliness.

Note: The ancient idea of the brow chakra suggesting the quality of the relationship between the individual and his or her mother obviously indicates a good relationship if the chakra is properly aligned, but a poor one if it is too strong or too weak. If it is too strong, the individual may behave badly to his or her mother, while if it is weak, the mother might hurt, use, or manipulate her child.

BODY AND HEALTH

Problems with the brow chakra lead to headaches, migraines, neuralgia, sinusitis, dizziness, or even a discombobulated feeling due to fatigue and shortage of sleep. Sleep can be disturbed during menopause, so it is no surprise to find that this chakra is connected to those hormonal problems that cause the sweating and bloating that disturb sleep.

The brow chakra rules the left eye, the pituitary gland, the central nervous system, the brain, and everything in the head, including tumors, strokes, blindness, and spinal difficulties. Needless to say, this chakra rules movement and coordination.

SPIRITUAL LINK

On a rather grand scale, the brow chakra is said to be one of the seats of the soul. It indicates the inner being and the source of creative energy. Some say it holds the *Akashic Records* and our experiences of past lives. It is said to hold the key to the soul's purpose in this lifetime. The brow chakra encourages people to look into what might exist in the rest of the universe, and to find the reason for our existence.

On a more down-to-earth level, the brow chakra relates to emotional intelligence and maturity, and it helps us to see what's behind our own actions and those of others. It brings the gifts of intuition and inspiration and it allows us to access messages from the spirit world. It is especially connected to clairvoyance and second sight.

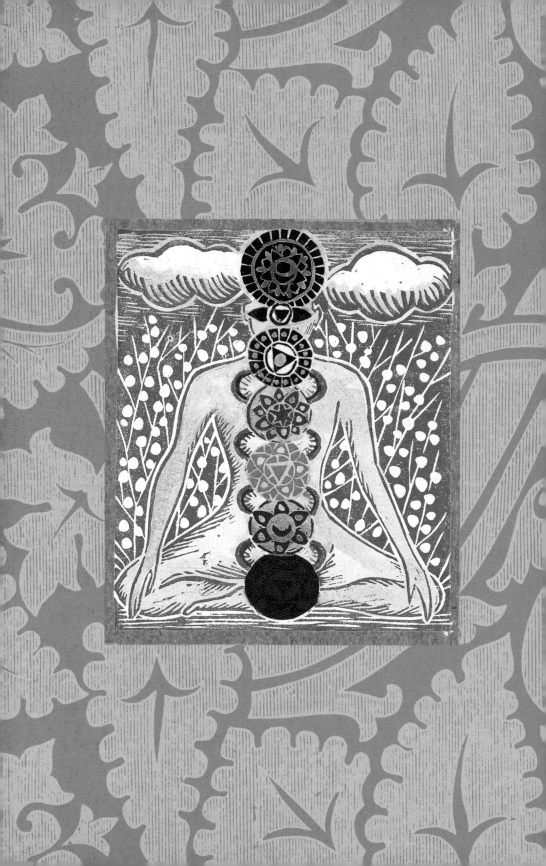

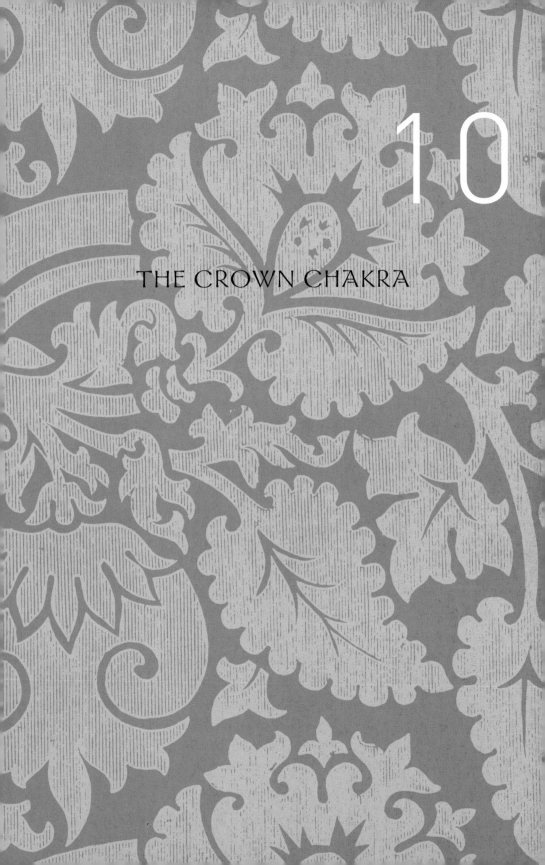

10

THE CROWN CHAKRA

Vedic name:	Sahasrara
Number:	The seventh chakra
Other names:	Violet chakra
Central concept:	Spirituality
Color:	Violet, purple; in some traditions, white or gold
Lotus petals:	Technically one thousand, but often shown as a purple lily
Shapes:	Lotus, lily
Element:	Light
Planet:	Saturn
Zodiac sign:	Capricorn
Health connection:	Head, central nervous system
Balance:	Ying/Yang; thus, masculine and feminine
Gland:	Pineal/Pituitary
Sense:	Oneness with the universe
Facial area:	Head
Mantra:	*Nnn*
Music:	Silence

LOCATION

The crown chakra is located at the top of the head, slightly to the back of it.

BASIC PURPOSE

The crown chakra is hard to define, and it is all too easy to descend into pseudospiritual waffle while attempting to do so—but I will do my best to keep things simple and straightforward.

Consider the idea of connectedness, and you are well on the way to understanding this chakra. For instance, it links all of us to everyone else on earth, so it suggests the idea of the brotherhood of man. It unites us with Heaven, the universe, and Spirit, but it also reaches down through the chakra system to connect us to the earth beneath our feet. Therefore, it rules the interconnectedness of everything. It symbolizes faith and trust, along with the ability to pray and to know that God will lead us in the right direction.

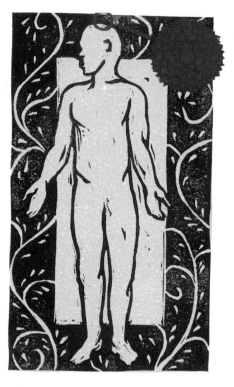

Crown Chakra

A person with a strong crown chakra looks forward to the future with optimism, and a strong crown chakra is also associated with joy, happiness, and peace of mind.

A STRONG CROWN CHAKRA

People with a strong crown chakra are idealistic and have a deep reverence for all forms of life. They are kindhearted and may be somewhat self-sacrificing. They can empathize with others to the extent that they almost feel their pain. They understand all types of people. They are highly intelligent.

This chakra contains memories of the past and of past lives but also some inkling of Heaven and the next life. This is the gateway to the higher consciousness, spirituality, guided intuition, and an understanding of the real meaning of life and of the afterlife. Those who have a strong crown chakra understand their purpose on earth and can see the best way forward. However, their values and their choice of pathway are spiritual rather than material, so they choose not to join the rat race. The crown chakra rules faith, trust, prayer, meditation, and wisdom. It also links to happiness, bliss, and moments of true ecstasy and joy. It brings a sense of balance and spiritual awareness.

Oddly enough, feelings of loneliness, isolation, bereavement, and absolute desolation can be linked to this chakra even when it is strong. The concept is not easy to grasp, but the idea is that when people are utterly lost, bereaved, betrayed, or unhappy, they are most likely to turn to prayer. It is at these times that they ask the age-old questions— "Why me?" "Why this?" "Why now?" It is then that they pray for the strength to cope with life. Misery turns people inward to contemplate the spiritual side of life, and this chakra is all about such inward journeys. Thus, in a strange way, awareness and growth of character can come out of heartbreak.

On a mundane level, those who have an abundance of strength in this chakra might choose a profession in which making a lot of money is not a priority, such as rabbi, nun, priest, social worker, or perhaps overseas aid worker. There is nothing written anywhere that says that this chakra is against someone earning money, but the individual should also possess a good soul. Indeed, those who work, earn money, and pay their bills have a sense of responsibility that denotes a strong crown chakra, but they never view money as the prime motivator.

Individuals with a strong crown chakra are ethical; they always try to do a good day's work in exchange for a good day's pay. If they sell something or perform a service, they are happy doing so if they believe that the product or service is of real benefit to others. These individuals can't stand people who take advantage, swindlers, and liars. They are honest and decent themselves, and they prefer to keep company with others who are equally honest and decent.

Note: Tradition suggests that the crown chakra carries memories of a father's love, along with feelings of sadness at having to grow up and leave him.

TOO MUCH CROWN CHAKRA

Too much crown chakra typifies those who are too involved with the world of Spirit to be able to function in the real world. These individuals need to become grounded. They may pray all the time. They take themselves very seriously, and they may be religious bores who have no ordinary interests and no other topics of conversation. They may have a judgmental and holier-than-thou attitude that makes others feel uncomfortable, and they consider themselves superior to those around them.

NOT ENOUGH CROWN CHAKRA

Some of those with a weak crown chakra are full of fears and phobias, so that they cannot enjoy life or look forward to the future with optimism. They fear death. If their lives are difficult, they find it hard to make changes, improve their situation, or move on. They have no faith in God or in the future, so they often feel blocked and unable to progress. They cannot pray, and they don't even try to access their own higher consciousness.

At worst, those who are lacking in crown chakra energy might be money minded, mundane, and earthly. At best, they may be wonderful moneymakers, and they probably value other people by measuring the money or possessions that they have. They may be completely taken up with the idea of wealth and possessions, so that they become materially rich but lack compassion or soul.

Often it takes loss, heartbreak, or bereavement for ordinary people to consider the soul, karma, the afterlife, and their purpose on earth, which is why severe distress is often the start of spiritual development.

Note: The connection with the father suggests that an overly strong or overly weak crown chakra is allied to a poor father-child relationship, where either the father is a bad parent or the child is bad to his or her father.

BODY AND HEALTH

The crown chakra rules the brain, especially the right side of it, and is also associated with the central nervous system. Thus, in individuals with a misaligned crown chakra there may be such problems as multiple sclerosis, schizophrenia, hallucinations, Parkinson's disease, epilepsy, Alzheimer's, bipolar disorder, or some other kind of severe mental disorder. This chakra also rules clinical depression.

Tradition suggests that the crown chakra rules the right eye, and such things as varicose veins and the skin. Thus, it is associated with rashes, eczema, warts, moles, bacteria, and probably also skin cancer.

SPIRITUAL LINK

Those who have a strong crown chakra are aware of their oneness and harmony with the universe and with all humankind. They are kind, gentle, and generous. They can see something good in the most difficult of people, and they have time for even the most unsavory or unwanted members of society. Needless to say, wealth and money don't attract them. Piling up wealth in Heaven is more their style.

Note: The crown chakra is the gateway to the spiritual world. Tradition says that the soul leaves the body via this chakra.

EXAMPLES OF INDIVIDUALS WITH STRONG CROWN CHAKRAS

Famous examples of people with strong crown chakras include Mahatma Gandhi, Mother Theresa, Pope John Paul II, and St. Francis of Assisi.

A less famous example of someone with a strong crown chakra was my friend Gordon Arthur Smith. Gordon was not a clever man or a great moneymaker; indeed, he ended his life living pretty much hand to mouth, but he had a hugely generous soul and a great deal of spiritual wisdom. He had little education and was not clever in the accepted sense, but where spiritual matters were concerned, he read widely and he traveled far and wide in search of answers to his many questions. If I ever needed the answer to a question of a spiritual nature, I could rely on Gordon to give me an answer that made perfect sense.

Gordon's advice to all seekers of the truth was to listen to everything and read everything, and then filter the information through one's own common sense before accepting something as undeniable truth. Good advice, indeed.

Another example is Vivien, who has always "been there" for

her family, friends, colleagues, and neighbors. People have only had to mention that they were putting on a fund-raising lunch for Viven to turn up with bowls of food; if they were sick, she was the first on the scene offering help. Her last job was managing an elder-care center where she was at everyone's beck and call. Yet Viven enjoyed being needed and doing what she felt was right. Vivien is now retired and enjoying her freedom, but she will still help those in need where she can. Vivien may not have much in the way of material goods, but she has a good karma.

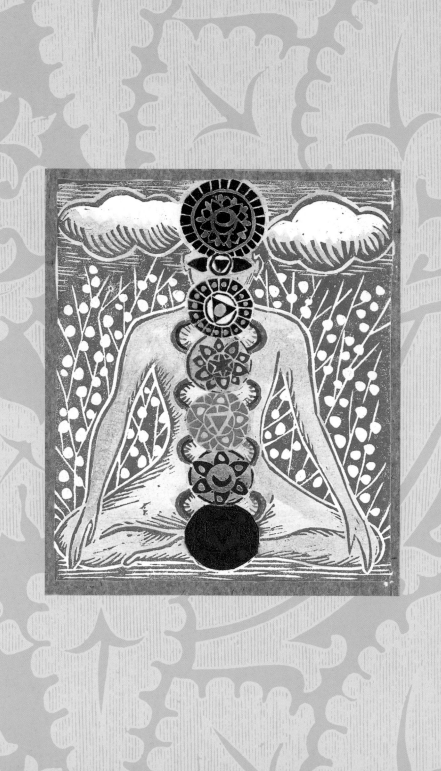

11

PHYSICAL CHAKRA HEALING

If you are unwell, please go to a conventional medical practitioner—visit your dentist, optician, podiatrist, or other relevant professional, as required. Once that process is in place, you can explore complementary therapies, which are ideal for some chronic ailments for which conventional medicine can do little; the same goes for some stress-related ailments. Other ailments need conventional medicine or even counseling and psychotherapy, but the process may be sped up or made easier by the use of complementary therapies or by spiritual healing. Nowadays, treatments that conventional doctors once laughed at are part of the establishment, with advertisements for them posted on hospital bulletin boards. Examples include osteopathy, chiropractors, aromatherapy, acupuncture, hypnotherapy, and reflexology. Some brow chakra ailments respond well to cranial-sacral osteopathy or zero balancing, which is a gentle form of massage and muscular manipulation.

If you are receiving conventional medical treatment, please remember to tell your doctor about any complementary treatment that you are also having, especially those that introduce substances into the body, such as homeopathy, herbal treatments, or aromatherapy.

SOME SIMPLE TECHNIQUES

Let us assume that you are a bit out of sorts and you feel that a boost to one of your chakras would make you feel better. Try this very simple and noninvasive method for rebalancing a slightly unsteady chakra. Take a piece of cloth or paper in the relevant chakra color and focus on the color. Breathe regularly and deeply for a while, as if you were taking the color into your body with each intake of breath.

Another simple and very pleasant form of chakra alignment is to add some fruits and vegetables of the appropriate color into your diet for a day or two. Don't just live on the one kind of food and exclude others; simply make sure that you include one item of its kind in your diet each day. Unbalanced eating can make you ill. For instance, if you eat too much citrus fruit or fruit juice, you can end up with cystitis and headaches, while too many carrots will turn your skin yellow! Here are some chakra-based suggestions for foods to help realign an off-kilter chakra:

Base chakra:	Tomatoes, red plums, straw-berries, raspberries
Sacral chakra:	Oranges, carrots, apricots, orange peppers
Solar plexus chakra:	Bananas, parsnips, yellow peppers, lemons, sweet corn
Heart chakra:	Green vegetables, apples, pears, gooseberries, kiwi
Throat chakra:	Plums, passion fruit, red grapes, blueberries
Brow chakra:	Blueberries, blackberries, black currants
Crown chakra:	Radishes, blackberries, black olives

It might seem strange to use color for healing, but it can have dramatic effects. About five or six hundred years ago, if a child became ill with chicken pox, the parents would give the child "the red treatment." This meant temporarily replacing the curtains and bedclothes in the child's room with ones made out of red material. It was believed that this weird therapy worked because something in the spectrum of the red color prevented chicken pox from forming scars. Similarly, bad cases of psoriasis can be treated by ultraviolet light, and some forms of psoriasis improve when exposed to sunlight, due to the ultraviolet rays in sunshine.

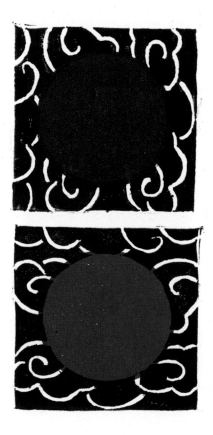

I think color is best used to change one's mood. When I am due to give a talk or a presentation, I instinctively choose to wear bright colors to give me confidence. If I need to be quiet and calm, I wear pale shades of blue, lavender, or cream. If you have trouble sleeping or relaxing, you should decorate your bedroom and living room in cool, quiet, pastel shades. If your child finds it hard to sleep, decorate his or her room in soft and neutral colors. People love to decorate children's rooms in very bright colors with Disney-type figures and patterns, and then they wonder why the poor kids can't sleep!

ALTAR HEALING

There are forms of healing that are noninvasive but very effective in their way, and for many of these, we can take ideas that come from religion as a whole and Wicca in particular. The following suggestions might help ease physical ailments, but they are particularly useful when helping someone who is unhappy or ill at ease.

Find a quiet spot in your house and put a small table in it. If you are short of space, a bookshelf or the top of a chest of drawers will do. Put a clean white cloth and a candleholder on your altar. Select the color that is appropriate to the chakra that you wish to heal; then place a piece of cloth or a paper napkin in that color on the altar. You can also use gems and stones of the appropriate type for a certain chakra. Add a candle or tea light in the relevant color. If you like, put a little dish with some appropriate essential oil on the altar, use an oil burner, or use an incense stick with an aroma that

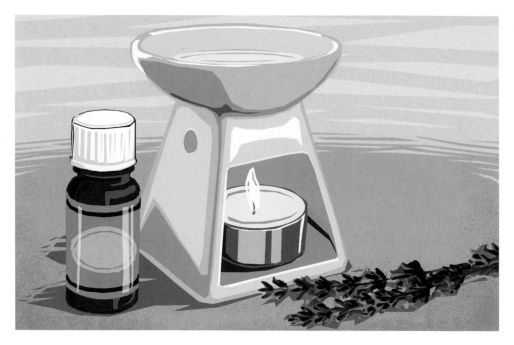

feels right for that chakra. You can put ribbons, buttons, beads, or anything else on the altar that you like and that happens to be the appropriate color.

Note: If you light candles or incense sticks, please stay in the room and keep an eye on them. Don't put candles, incense sticks or burners in a drafty area where they might fall over and cause a fire.

If you are giving healing to yourself, put a photograph of yourself on the altar; if you are giving healing to someone else, use his or her photo. If you have a particular piece of jewelry or other item that means a lot to you, you can add that, along with anything else that might be appropriate to you. The same goes for things that are appropriate to your friend or for things that relate to the ailment or the problem.

Even writing the concern or problem down on a piece of paper and putting that on the altar will help. For example, if someone is worried about a hospital appointment or an upcoming exam, they could put the letter about this on the altar. Once again, I remind you never to leave lighted candles, burners, or incense sticks unattended.

GEMSTONES AND METALS

A very nice form of energy healing is to use gems and other materials directly on the chakras. For this, you need to have your "patient" lie down, and then place stones or pieces of metal on the various chakras, as this will boost the healing energy. Where the base chakra is concerned, you might prefer to place the stone or metal on the person's legs, just above the knees, than in the traditional base chakra position. The choice of stones and metals is pretty large, and opinions vary as to which should be used where, as some are assigned to more than one chakra. As always, do what feels right to you.

CLEANSING AND ENERGIZING

Before you use any crystals, stones, metals, or other items, you should take the following steps:

- Collect some rainwater and wash the stones in it.
- Leave the stones to dry outside in the sunlight or on a sunny windowsill.

- Lay the stones on a clean cloth and imagine white light coming down on them from the universe; ask for the stones to help those who are in need of healing or relief from mental stress.
- Put the stones in a nice bag or box and keep them out of harm's way until you want to use them.
- Keep all objects that are used for spiritual purposes on a shelf above head height, in order to keep them closer to Heaven.

WHICH CRYSTALS TO USE ON WHICH CHAKRAS

The following lists show some of the stones or metals that you might choose as a healing boost for each chakra.

Base Chakra

- Black onyx
- Garnet
- Hematite
- Jasper
- Pyrite
- Ruby
- Obsidian
- Flint
- Iron

Sacral Chakra

- Amber
- Aventurine
- Carnelian
- Citrine
- Tiger's-eye
- Coral
- Jasper
- Moonstone
- Fire opal
- Topaz
- Silver

Solar Plexus Chakra

- Amber
- Amethyst
- Calcite
- Citrine
- Sodalite
- Tiger's-eye
- Topaz
- Gold

Heart Chakra

- Aventurine
- Emerald
- Jade
- Chrysocolla
- Agate
- Peridot
- Rose quartz
- Malachite
- Moonstone
- Pink tourmaline
- Green tourmaline
- Copper

Throat Chakra

- Turquoise
- Aquamarine
- Lapis lazuli
- Blue lace agate
- Sodalite
- Amazonite
- Celestine
- Fluorite
- Sapphire
- Cinnabar

Brow Chakra

- Clear quartz
- Lapis lazuli
- Amethyst
- Azurite
- Calcite
- Sapphire
- Fluorite
- Tin

Crown Chakra

- Diamond
- Zircon
- Amethyst
- Pearl
- Clear quartz
- Rose quartz
- Lead

ESSENTIAL OILS

It is always advisable to consult a qualified aromatherapist for the best treatment, because oils can have a profound effect on the body. It is better not to use these on the skin of someone who is seriously ill or who is taking other medication. There are special burners for use with essential oils that will waft the essence around the room, which is better than putting it directly on the skin. Please ask a qualified person to show you how to use the burner safely rather than experimenting with it. If you understand the principles of aromatherapy and can safely use oils on your client's skin, always dilute the oil with a suitable carrier oil.

Base Chakra

- Oak moss
- Patchouli
- Vetiver

Sacral Chakra

- Clary sage
- Jasmine
- Cinnamon
- Rose
- Citrus

Solar Plexus

- Bergamot
- Geranium
- Ginger
- Grapefruit
- Juniper
- Lemon
- Peppermint
- Rosemary

Heart Chakra

- Bergamot
- Rose
- Ylang-ylang
- Lemongrass

Throat Chakra

- Rosemary
- Chamomile
- Frankincense
- Sandalwood
- Geranium

Brow Chakra

- Lavender
- Hyacinth
- Geranium
- Pine
- Sage
- Rose

Crown Chakra

- Frankincense
- Myrrh
- Sandalwood
- Bay
- Lavender
- Valerian
- Jasmine

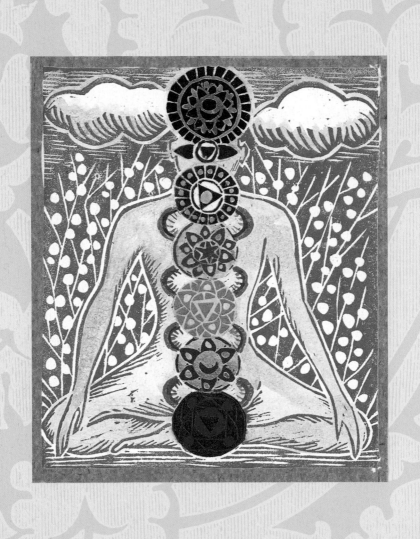

12

EMOTIONAL OR MENTAL
CHAKRA HEALING

There are thousands of emotional and psychological situations that plague us, but we can focus on only a few obvious ones in this book. Let us look at some scenarios that typify the problems attached to each chakra and see what sensible steps you can take to help yourself.

BASE CHAKRA

The base chakra is about survival, so at the most fundamental level, this means having enough clean water, food, clothing, shelter, and appropriate medicines to stay alive and healthy. To give yourself mental healing surrounding this issue, pose a comparison between your own life, with all its ups and downs, and that of someone who is stuck in a refugee camp in Africa, or wandering around in a state of shock following a natural disaster. In more mundane terms, to address issues surrounding the base chakra, it is wise to avoid back alleys, dangerous areas, and shortcuts and to avoid taking part in improperly supervised extreme sports. In emotional terms, being on the receiving end of sustained bullying is not good for your mental health.

Where physical or mental danger is concerned, your best bet is to get yourself out of that situation quickly, even if it means moving away from a particular area or dumping harmful friends and relatives. If you are at a social event and someone bothers you, excuse yourself for a bathroom visit; while you're there, call a cab and go home. Do this even if you have a partner or friends at the event; just tell them you have a migraine and explain the real reason for your departure later—if you even feel that's necessary. Never accept a ride home from a strange person.

Give yourself spiritual sustenance by doing the things that make you happy, such as singing, dancing, swimming, playing sports, and having fun. Sports, energetic activities, and dancing are particularly attuned to the base chakra. Alternatively, calm the chakra by meditating and daydreaming. When you have some time to yourself, sit or lie down, close your eyes, and imagine white light that is flecked with healing turquoise or pale blue coming down and flooding your body. Let this light focus most of its energy on the base chakra.

Realize your limitations and forgive yourself when you discover that you can't do everything to perfection. Take a rest from time to time.

SACRAL CHAKRA

The sacral chakra rules relationships and everything that can happen within them. This chakra rules gut feelings, and yours will tell you the truth if you listen to them with honesty, so listen to your inner voice and trust your own instincts. Filter everything through your own intellect. Don't allow yourself to be railroaded into anything, whether it is sex, giving money or support to someone, or allowing someone to "crash" in your home. Don't turn your back on your friends and family just because you think you have found your soul mate. If your lover becomes jealous of the time you spend with friends and family, this is a warning sign of potential future abuse.

Remind yourself that you can't possibly be responsible for everything that goes wrong in your life. You don't have enough power for that. Unpleasant things happen to all of us from time to time. It's just the way things are.

SOLAR PLEXUS CHAKRA

The solar plexus chakra rules self-esteem, self-respect, and personal power. If this chakra is misaligned, others might push you around, or you might behave in a controlling or bullying manner. Aim for a happy medium: Don't shrink from the challenges of life, but don't hurt others either. Look after your diet and health, get some exercise, drink plenty of water, and eat properly. This will make you feel better, so that you become strong enough to fight off moments of despair. If people take advantage of you, stand in front of a mirror and practice saying no. Walk around your house or yard with your hand in a "stop" position and say, "Don't you dare take advantage of me!" If you can do this in a safe situation, you might just be able to do it when you need to.

If you are jealous of people who have money, status, or a better lifestyle than you do, try envying the queen of England, because she has everything, and that will save you the bother of having to envy everyone between your level and hers. If you feel jealous of love rivals or if you yearn for someone who doesn't love you, use a meditation to envision some way of cutting yourself away from the painful situation or letting it go. Then take yourself off to fresh woods and pastures new. You may find new friends who appreciate you when you are in a new environment.

There are many meditations for getting rid of things. Try this one, for example: Sit down quietly and open your chakras. Imagine a large plastic bag and see yourself holding the handles of the bag. Imagine the other person, the problem, or your feelings about the situation going into the bag. When the bag is full, tie it up, put it into a garbage can, and then imagine yourself cutting the handles or letting them go. Wave good-bye to the bag of trouble.

HEART CHAKRA

The heart chakra concerns love and relationships. If your heart chakra is misaligned, love can make the world go wrong! Love, self-sacrifice, and affection are wonderful, and it is great to be kind, loving, and giving, but not if you constantly choose unkind, unloving takers as partners. On the contrary, you may be too choosy and demanding for anyone to be able to stand your company for long. There are many courses that teach awareness, so why not take a few of them? Learn how to respect yourself and love yourself, because then you will attract the respect and love of others.

If a love relationship starts well but becomes untenable, then accept that you might have to call it a day. If you lie to yourself or to others, or if you are constantly lied to, try to figure out why this is happening. For instance, is this just a case of a few little white lies that are designed to save unnecessary friction, or are you frightened of your partner? Be honest with yourself.

THROAT CHAKRA

The throat chakra is the chakra of communication—or the lack of it! Lynne Lauren is a professional psychic who runs workshops, and she says that this is the chakra that most people have trouble with and it is often the one with the greatest need for healing.

This chakra is associated with a host of communication problems, such as not speaking up when something bothers you or not letting others know how you really feel. Alternatively, you might be too quick to express unpleasant opinions or inclined to blurt out remarks that you instantly regret. You may fuss about unimportant matters or you may never say what you really mean. These are just a few of the many problems people have in communicating their own needs and feelings.

BROW CHAKRA

The brow chakra rules excellence in behavior, faithfulness, courage, and truthfulness. It rules confidence in one's abilities, a realistic sense of one's own value, and a sense of purpose. Chakra treatment to this area can help people to become more able and more confident. It can also aid the development of intuition, sensitivity, and the ability to channel or link to Spirit. There isn't much to say about the brow or crown chakras, because they are only really put to use for such things as intuition, the use of psychic gifts, prayer, and the ability to obtain spiritual guidance.

CROWN CHAKRA

The crown chakra rules the link to Spirit and the first slight glimmering of the next world. This chakra will need healing if a person is too interested in religion and spiritual matters for common sense to apply.

OTHER CHAKRAS

As you will see in the next chapter, there are many other chakras, and if one happens to connect with a body area that is sore—such as a hand or knee—some healing directed into it can do no harm.

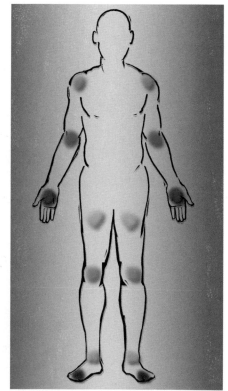

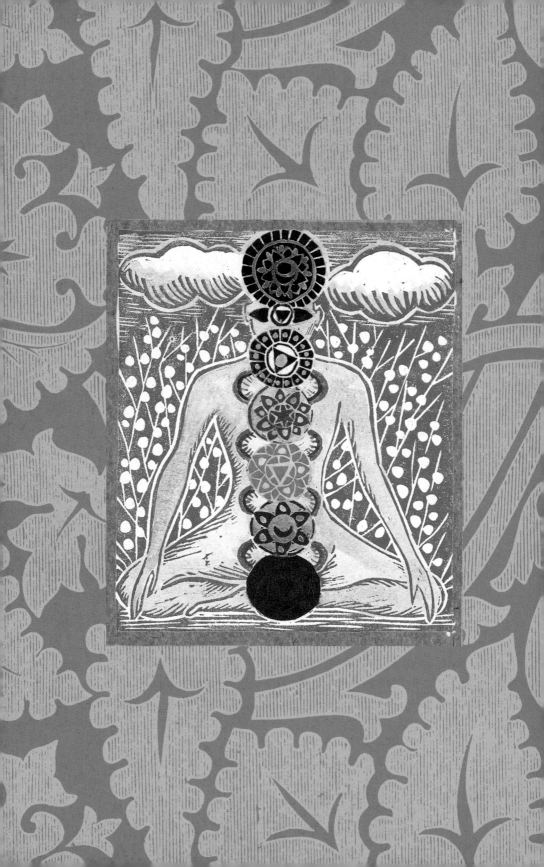

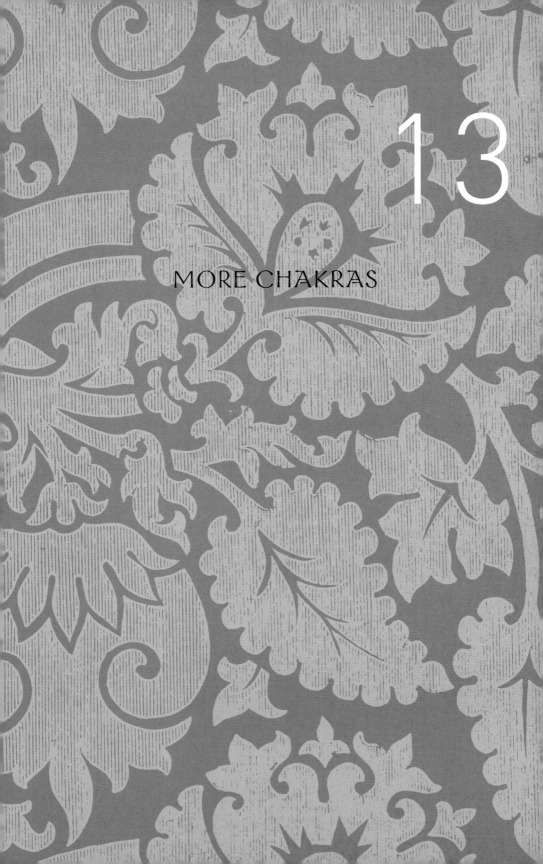

13

MORE CHAKRAS

When it comes to the extra chakras, there are a lot to choose from and many different ideas as to what they might be used for. Some are well-known, but others are still subject to ongoing discussion among spiritual people.

REMEMBER WHERE CHAKRAS ARE

An easy way of keeping a record of the chakras in your own body is to dig out a photo that shows you standing up and wearing fitted clothes such as jeans and a T-shirt. Make a few photocopies, and use these to draw the chakras as you discover them. When you have found all the chakras you want to use, make a nice, neat copy, indicate the chakras in colors that you think are suitable, and then laminate the final picture. My experience has shown that, over time, you will become aware of another six or eight chakras in addition to the basic seven.

Awareness of additional chakras can come through reading books, finding information on the Internet, or talking to healers and psychics, but it can also come through use and common sense. For example, you might suddenly realize that you habitually rub or scratch a particular part of your body when you are doing spiritual work. You may rub another area when you are agitated or some other part of the body when you are particularly happy, and yet another area will bother you when you are thinking deeply.

Often there are chakras on either side of the body that mirror each other. For example, there are two on either side of the spine, below the shoulder blades; these are linked to higher learning. If you want to put your mind to something deep or difficult, it might be worth focusing your mind on them for a moment or two, so that they open for you.

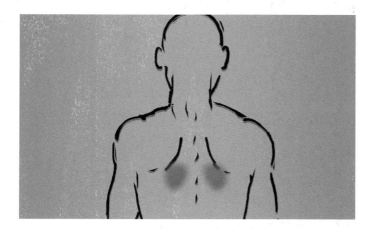

Similarly, if you want to feel more confident, focus your mind on the chakras on either side of your pelvic area. Give them a surreptitious rub if it is convenient to do so.

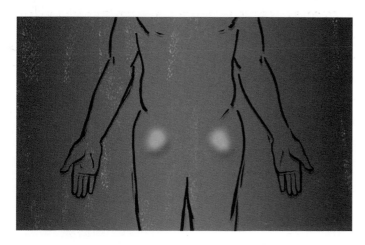

THE HANDS AND ARMS

Every healer and many other psychics are aware that each hand has a chakra that runs right through it from the back of the hand to the palm.

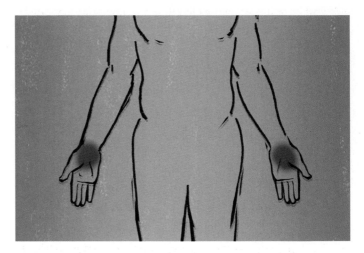

These chakras are useful when giving healing, when you wish to feel someone's or something's aura, or when you want to give a massage. They will help with anything that you need to do with your hands—even something as ordinary as hairdressing!

If you want to feel these chakras at work, try this exercise:

- Put your hands together in front of you.
- Part your hands to about eighteen inches.
- Slowly bring them back together.
- Stop when you feel a slight pressure, as if the air between your hands has become thicker.

If nothing happens, try this: Hold your hands out in front of you with one palm facing upward and the other downward, with a gap of about three or four inches between them. Then swap them around so that you change the hands that are facing up and down. Keep on swapping them until your arms feel tired. If you don't get much of a reaction from your own body alone, try this with someone else so that each of you has a palm that faces the other.

FINGERS

Each fingertip has a little chakra of its own. If you want to see these in action, take a pendulum or use a pendant on a chain and hold this over your fingers, one at a time. The pendulum will move in a different direction over each finger. If you don't get any reaction, try working on someone else's hands, because the interaction between you might make it work more successfully than doing it on yourself alone. In practical terms, these chakras also help when giving healing or any kind of hands-on treatment.

FOOT CHAKRAS

Foot chakras go through the insteps and out through the soles of the feet.

The foot chakras help you to ground yourself, so if you have been doing too much meditation or psychic or spiritual work

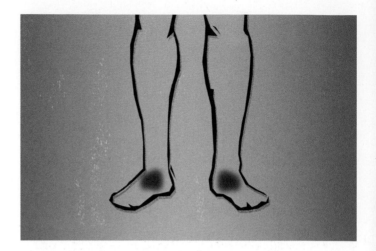

and you feel light-headed and spacey, or if you have a headache, try to get outdoors, and stand or walk on the earth or on grass with bare feet for a few moments. Be careful not to cut or hurt your feet. These chakras link you to Mother Earth and help you to regain a sense of proportion. You might even like to extend some imaginary light from your body, down through your feet to the earth below. This is a calming exercise.

ELBOW CHAKRAS

The elbows have chakras, but opinion varies as to whether these are shining out on the points of the elbows or going through them from side to side like rivets. Some people find that techniques that use the hands, elbows, and shoulders encourage those chakras to open. A typical example would be when doing aromatherapy.

SHOULDER CHAKRAS

The shoulders have chakras; they run through the outer part of the shoulders, from front to back.

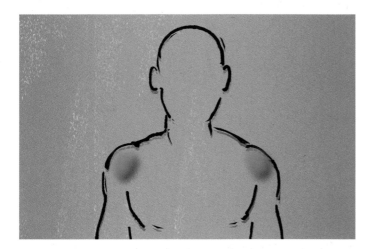

I feel my shoulder chakras opening whenever I do anything of a psychic or spiritual nature. Interestingly, some books on chakras show the shoulder chakras as being in the armpit area, but mine aren't. They definitely run through the shoulders from the back of my body to the front, just below the area where a shoulder pad in a coat would sit.

THE EIGHTH CHAKRA

The eighth chakra sits above the head and is often depicted as a white glow or a white flower. I think this is where the confusion surrounding the color of the crown chakra arises. Some feel that it should be colored purple and others say white. My view is that the crown chakra is purple but that the eighth chakra, which sits above the crown chakra, is white.

Tradition says that at the time of death, the soul leaves the body through a small hole in the top of the head, and the eighth chakra is the last link between the human world and all our bodily concerns, and the world of Spirit. It contains karmic residue that is taken into the first stages of the afterlife.

Not everyone agrees with this image; many psychics report the spiritual body parting the physical one via an umbilical cord.

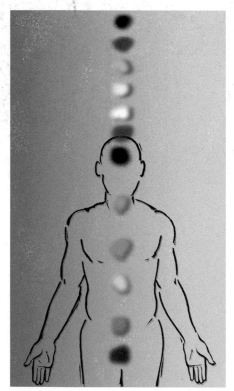

THE HIGHER CHAKRAS

Hindu tradition suggests that the eighth chakra is topped by another four chakras that line up above the head, with the last one being situated about two feet above the head. It is said that each of these has a different spiritual purpose.

DOUBLED CHAKRAS

To discuss the doubled chakras, we must return to the seven major chakras, but we now take a closer look at two of them. The doubled chakras are the heart chakra and the brow chakra. Some Hindu illustrations show these doubled chakras as one slightly above the other.

Doubled Heart Chakra

Both heart chakras deal with love, but the lower one is said to rule earthly, romantic love, and the love of a child, a family member, a friend, or even a pet. This chakra can even be associated with obsessive love, although that is also strongly influenced by the base and sacral chakras. The upper heart chakra is aligned to the love of God.

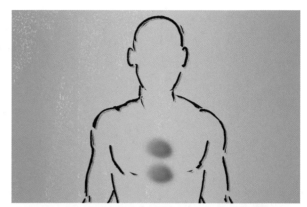

Doubled Brow Chakra

The lower brow chakra is between and slightly above the

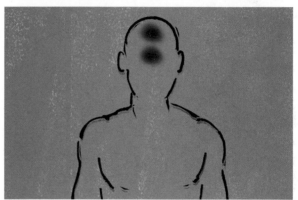

level of the eyes, and this chakra concerns the activities of the mind and the thinking process. The upper brow chakra is in the middle of the forehead and is linked to mercy, gentleness, and empathy.

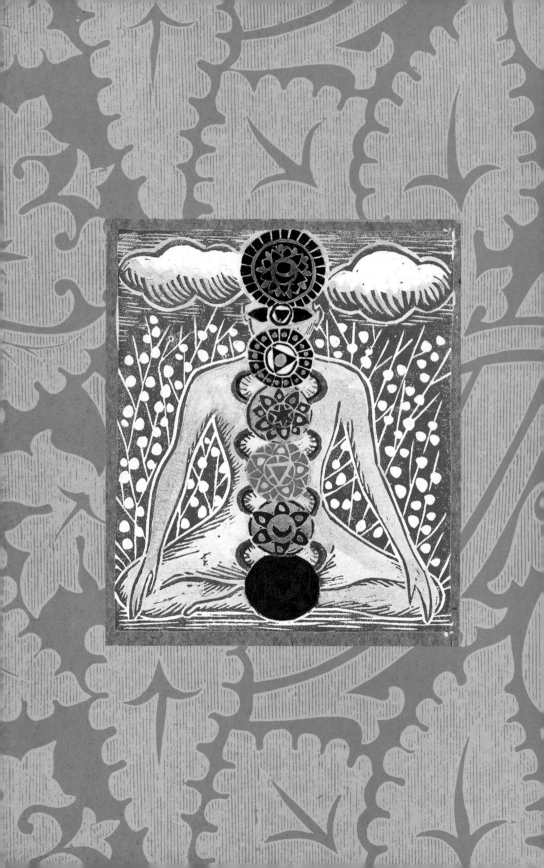

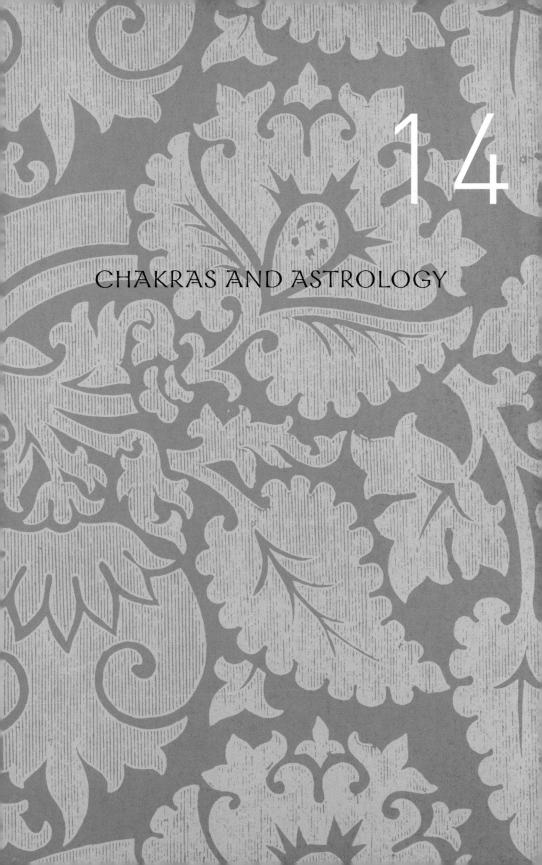

14

CHAKRAS AND ASTROLOGY

If you are into astrology, the connections between the chakras and the Sun, the Moon, and the ascendant are fascinating, and you will soon be able to pick out thóse that are strong on your birth chart. If you know the signs occupied by your other planets, descendant, medium coeli and immum coeli, and if you know which are well or badly aspected, you can fill in even more gaps. Here are the ancient connections:

Chakras, the Zodiac, and the Planets

Chakra	Zodiac Signs	Planet
Base	Aries, Scorpio	Mars
Sacral	Cancer	Moon
Solar plexus	Leo	Sun
Heart	Taurus, Libra	Venus
Throat	Gemini, Virgo	Mercury
Brow	Sagittarius, Pisces	Jupiter
Crown	Capricorn, Aquarius	Saturn

Astrology is not an exact science, and people differ in the way they express the various parts of their birth chart, but the following is the standard interpretation. Your Sun sign represents your basic personality. Your Moon sign represents your inner personality, and it is often linked to the way you relate or react to others. It is concerned with your emotions and feelings, and it can reveal your real motives, needs, and feelings about life, which you might keep hidden from others for safety's sake. The rising sign often relates to what you do and the way you act in the outside world, partly at least, because it represents the programming that you received when you were young.

Example: Lily

Lily was born with the Sun in Leo, the Moon in Gemini, and Cancer rising. Lily is a warmhearted person who is extremely loyal to those she loves, and she is also a hard worker (Sun in Leo; solar plexus chakra). She works in the travel trade, she is on the phone a lot, and she works on a computer. She is also extremely fond of her brother and of his family (Moon in Gemini; throat chakra). She loves her beautifully decorated home; she also loves to travel and take vacations; and her family means a lot to her (Cancer rising; sacral chakra).

Lily was born with severe problems in her reproductive system and cannot have children (sacral chakra). She has hypoglycemia, and there is a lot of diabetes in her family (solar plexus chakra), so she may well develop it later in life. She suffers from throat problems and gets bronchitis after a cold (throat chakra).

Lily is well thought of at work and is often promoted to senior positions (solar plexus chakra), but she isn't really that ambitious and sometimes finds this a burden, as people and stress get her down (sacral chakra). She listens to people and deals with them all day long, so she just wants to switch off from it all when she gets home. Her husband and family lean on her, so she doesn't always get the chance. She is practical but also intuitive, and she can see and feel her way around problems and work toward long-term goals (throat chakra).

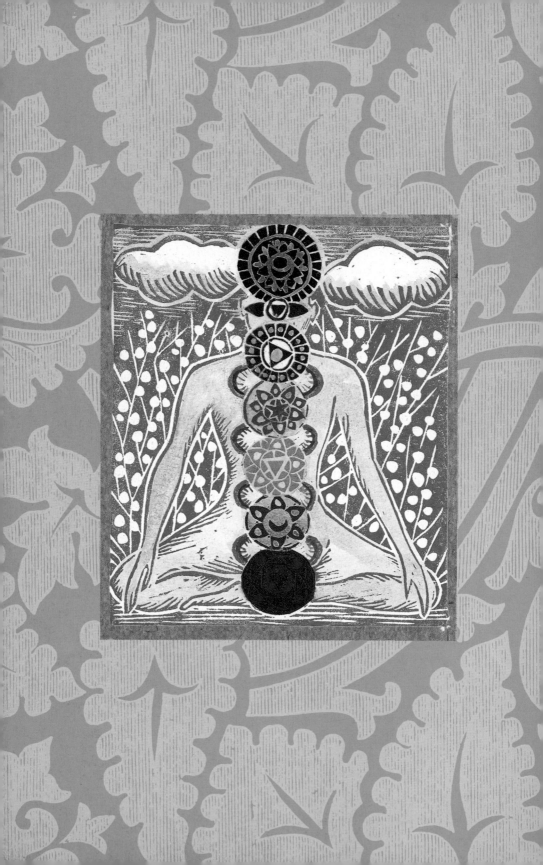

15

KUNDALINI

Kundalini is a force or energy that rises up through the chakra system from base to crown. Traditional illustrations depict kundalini as a snake that snoozes at the base of the body until something wakes it up, upon which it uncurls and rises up through the chakra system.

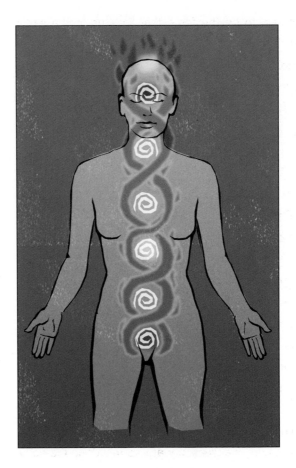

The chakras revolve in alternate directions, which is why some people see them as cogs in a wheel.

I prefer to think of kundalini as white smoke rising upward from a fire and passing by the revolving drums of the chakras rather than as a snake uncurling. Perhaps it is just that our culture is not too keen on snakes, or maybe I object to the idea of my body being inhabited by one.

Kundalini is said to be the force that links us to the earth beneath our feet and the heavens above our heads. It brings sudden enlightenment, and it can bring feelings of ecstasy of the kind that people experience when performing certain shamanic rituals. It can be activated by doing yoga and by meditating, and of course by opening the chakras and focusing on it.

Another way of raising kundalini is by having sex. When one experiences an especially powerful orgasm, it is not uncommon to see colors swirling around in one's head for a few moments afterward; this is part of the kundalini effect. When too much kundalini rushes to the head, or when it arrives there too quickly, you can feel spacey or you can get a headache. Have you ever developed a nasty headache after very good sex? If so, the kundalini force is responsible. The way to ease this effect is to open the crown chakra so that the kundalini force is set free to reach the heavens.

Your kundalini force can give you a headache after doing spiritual work. The cure is a glass of water to rehydrate the body and, if necessary, a couple of painkillers.

conclusion

So now we have taken a look at the chakra system, explored the seven major chakras in detail, and looked briefly into some others. We have discovered some ways of healing the emotional, mental, physical, and spiritual problems that arise when chakras are blocked, misaligned, or too open. You can ease these problems with energy healing or crystal healing and by using appropriate complementary therapies, along with conventional medicine when it is needed. Now it is time for you to use your chakras in any way that you care to, but remember to shut them again after doing any spiritual work, or you will feel invaded by unwanted energies and you will find it hard to sleep.

Good luck!

index